Alicia's Updates

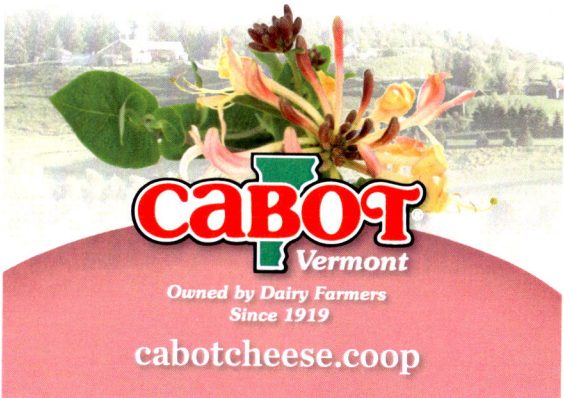

Alicia's Updates

A Mother's Memoir of Pediatric Cancer

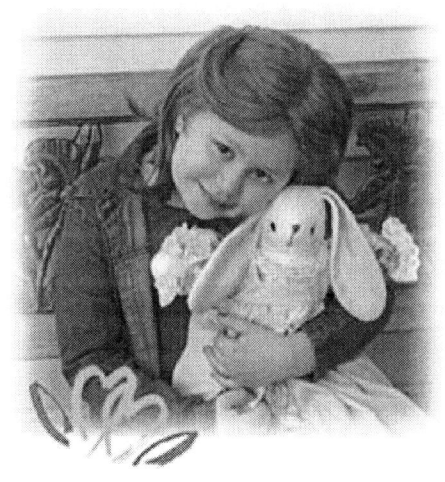

Rene A. Fesler

A portion of the proceeds from this book are being donated to the Honeysuckle Foundation
for Children with Cancer (www.honeysucklefoundation.org), the not for profit foundation
founded by Rene and Alicia during Alicia's illness.

This book was printed in the United States of America.

To order additional copies of this book, contact:
Xlibris Corporation
1-888-795-4274
www.Xlibris.com
Orders@Xlibris.com
47041

CONTENTS

Preface...9

Beginnings 11
A Bit About Me...13
Cancer..14
A Parent Myself...16
"Mommy, My Back Hurts" 17
Too Much Information 18
Dr. John Figures It Out 19
All About Alicia...22
Polly Pockets To The Rescue...23
The Emergency Room 24
Needles And Other Scary Stuff..26
Other Obligations..27
Parenting By "Moi" 28
Relief..29
Preparing For Surgery..30
Surgery Day, Thursday, January 17....................................31
A Time To Cry 33
Hospital Life 35
There Is No Place Like Home 36
Alicia Updates 37
Mommy, I Don't Want To Lose My Hair 39
Cancer MAkes You Either Bitter Or Better........................41
Things Go Ponder 43
Grandparents The "Other" Parents 46
Let People Help...51
Nursing For The Non-Nursing Types 101 56
The Power Of People 57
Cancer Education For Kids 59
"This Is The Operator Calling" 66
Comfortable In Your Own Skin 70

I Am Tired And Don't Want To Do This Anymore 79
Life's Little Treasures...81
Nurses And Doctors Are Your Friends 88
Statistics And Other Things That Just Don't Make Sense 96
Some Things Are Beyond Our Control 97
Life Is Not Fair 118
What My Friends Have Learned 139
Life After Cancer..170

Index..173

To my daughters,
Alicia, who is my inspiration, and Lauren,
who is my motivation.

PREFACE

THIS BOOK STARTED as a group of e-mails—a way to communicate with my family and friends during a family crisis in a high-tech way. Rather than call everyone on the telephone to keep them updated on Alicia's progress, it was easier to send an e-mail. The list of recipients grew as well as the e-mails. The content started as strictly informational and grew to be inspirational. Writing was effortless, and the words seemed to flow as the circumstances surrounding us changed daily. I found writing these very therapeutic. I would write them and then hit send. Friends responded, and some even forwarded my e-mails to their friends. Many people encouraged me to publish these. My aspirations for publishing came a few years after Alicia's treatment around 2007. I finally sat down and read what I had written years before. I laughed, I cried, and I realized just how lucky and blessed we are. We took a situation that was overwhelming and hard to bear and turned it into an experience of a lifetime. Our journey had many passengers as everyone around us was soon involved in our lives and the life of Alicia. Through this experience, a foundation was born, and many more lives were touched. The Honeysuckle Foundation for Children with Cancer *(www.honeysucklefoundation.org)* started because of what lies within these pages. My philosophy of quality of life being just as important as the quantity of days was the model for our mission and the message of our story. This book is written for everyone who has faced adversity and for those who have not. It is written as a message of hope and living life to the fullest. My hope is that anyone who reads our story will enjoy it and realize that each day is a gift. There are no guarantees for tomorrow, so make the most of what you have today and never forget to be thankful for what you do have.

BEGINNINGS

MY NAME IS Rene, and I am no one special. I have been a stay-at-home mom for nineteen years and have loved every minute of it. *Well, maybe not every minute,* but most. I have three incredible children. Lauren, the eldest, is a bright, focused, and a beautiful young woman whom I admire for her convictions and her maturity. J. J., the only boy, suffers from middle-child syndrome, throwing that phrase at me or his sisters whenever something doesn't go his way. He is a smart and sensitive young man who is quick to laugh, quick to cry, and quick to love. Alicia, the youngest, is typical of most babies in a family. She is spoiled, in a good way, doted upon, and the apple of her family's eye, including her siblings. She too is a special young girl who brings a unique meaning to the words *compassion* and *empathy*—an inspiration to me. My children are my pride and joy—my motivation to get up in the morning and the reason I need to go to sleep so early at night. My devotion to them and my family has been my sole focus and purpose for my entire adult life. It actually is quite nice to be average. Average means you are like everyone else. Your problems, trials, and tribulations are much like those of the rest of the world: kids not doing their homework, an appliance or car that breaks down, and infighting among the relatives. These problems—that while to most people may seem overwhelming and the cause of much stress—are actually beautifully simple. The reality is, however, we usually can't recognize the beautiful simplicity of our problems when we are overwhelmed by them.

A BIT ABOUT ME

WHEN I WAS a youngster, I dreamt of growing up and doing something wonderful or exceptional one day. A pilot, an author, or an archeologist were some of the various professions I would dream about. These professions were exciting and intriguing to me. The choices changed weekly, but the possibilities seemed endless. I wanted to be important. I wanted to have an impact on others' lives, and I wanted people to know it. My belief at that time was my importance in this world needed to be measured in the amount of recognition I would receive. Whether it would be accolades from a boss, a raise in pay, or notoriety, I would be able to measure my success in these tangible things. As I soon learned, however, we plan and God laughs. My life would not be as glamorous or as wonderful as I had dreamt of during my childhood; however, it would be very fulfilling. Securing a bachelors degree in management and communications, I settled into an administrative job, got married, and was enjoying my life for what it was—a life much like everyone else's life that I knew. I was happy, and life was good. With the birth of my eldest daughter, Lauren, I would become the thing I found the most rewarding—a stay-at-home mom. My future for the next fourteen years would be filled with diapers, playdates, homework, and carpooling. Fights between the siblings, holidays, school concerts, and the never-ending list of what Moms do for their kids. The hardest job in the world, I was the twenty-four-hour-seven-day-a-week caregiver for my children—the stay-at-home mom who did it all from child rearing to house painting to gardening. I did numerous things that kept me busy from early in the morning until late at night, and while complaining from time to time, I was enjoying every moment of it. I was doing something I loved to do, I was a mom. One by one, my children arrived until there were three, adding more work and chaos and more love and enjoyment to my life. A suburban housewife, I relished my role, and I loved my average life—a place of comfort and contentment. All of that changed on January 17, 2002. That was the day my youngest daughter Alicia was diagnosed with cancer.

CANCER

CANCER IS SCARY. I don't care who you are, where you live, or what socioeconomic group you belong to. The word *cancer* strikes fear in the hearts of all—an automatic thought of death and a word no one ever wants to hear, especially when you are talking about a child, your child. Being a middle-aged woman, I grew up in the era if a friend, relative, or acquaintance was diagnosed with this insidious disease, people were horrified and grew silent when hearing the news. No one spoke about it, tried to understand it, and certainly didn't embrace those who were afflicted by it. The thought process was, those with cancer were going to die. Some people actually believed you could *catch* cancer, much like a cold. In order to protect yourself and your own health, you needed to avoid cancer patients. Then there were those people who just couldn't *deal* with the horror of it and did not and could not handle watching a friend or loved one struggle with treatment to only possibly die. I remember when I was a young girl of twelve a family friend's daughter was battling leukemia. Joann was a pretty and a vivacious twelve-year-old, who, other than her bald head with a bandana on top of it, seemed very much like me. My parents were friends with her family, and both our families encouraged the friendship between Joann and me. While no one hid from me the fact that Joann was fighting for her life, everyone supported and helped nurture our friendship through playdates and telephone contact. I enjoyed Joann's company immensely and looked forward to our time together that was filled with usual childhood pranks and nonsense. Teasing our brothers, playing hide-and-seek, and experimenting with makeup and nail polish. I learned all too quickly, however, about the cold hand of death that cancer grasps with when Joann, my childhood friend, lost her battle to leukemia at the young age of thirteen. The overwhelming feeling of sadness I felt at the time seemed insurmountable as I tried to understand how my then thirteen-year-old friend could die. I felt sad for the loss of my friend, I felt sad for all she had been through just to eventually lose out to her cancer, and I felt sad that her parents, as well as the other adults helping her, were not able to save her, and I felt sad to now learn the cruelest lesson in life firsthand: some kids die. Life was not fair, and this just proved to me how unfair it was. My memories of Joann, while filled with laughter and fun, were also a cruel lesson to a then thirteen-year-old that some things in this life are beyond anyone's control. As much as we believe we are in control of our destiny, our children's lives, and the world around us, we are not. In fact most things in our lives we have absolutely no control over, these are the things in God's hands.

A PARENT MYSELF

FAST FORWARD ALMOST thirty years from Joann's death. I am now a parent with young children; the furthest thing from my mind, as is with most parents, was pediatric cancer. A few years before Alicia was born, my family went to Disney World, with Lauren and J. J. in tow. We were there to have fun, go on rides, and enjoy ourselves on a wonderful vacation. Getting off one of the rides one day, I remember seeing a bald, frail, young girl sitting in a wheelchair. Her parents were pushing her in her chair down to the handicap-accessible entrance to carry her onto the ride that my children and I just got off. I stared at those parents and their little girl and a lump grew in my throat and tears welled up in my eyes. I made my own assumption as to what was wrong. She looked like she had cancer. Typical emaciated dark-skinned look, sunken eyes, and such weakness she could not walk. I walked away from that ride holding my children's hands even tighter as I was feeling overwhelmed with sorrow and sick to my stomach. My thoughts at that moment were brought back to my friend Joann and the struggle that her parents faced. I couldn't help but try and imagine what this family's lives were like. For the rest of that day in Disney World, one of the happiest places on earth, I was overwhelmed with a sense of dread and heartache after witnessing a sick child. Little did I know at that time that I would find out firsthand just how difficult life could be when your child is sick. A few short years later with the words spoken by a pediatric neurosurgeon, "Alicia has cancer," I was now going to find out how Joann's parents and how the parents of the girl in Disney World and countless other parents around the world feel, when they are told their child has cancer. So how did we get to this point? What happened that brought a then six-year-old little girl into surgery on that fateful day to have a surgeon give us such horrible news? As with any story, there is a beginning, and ours began with Alicia and a bad backache.

"MOMMY, MY BACK HURTS"

M OTHERS KNOW THEIR children. We have an uncanny ability to sense when they are not telling the truth, when they are happy or sad, and, more importantly, we know when they are sick. When Alicia first got sick in December of 2001, I had an uncomfortable feeling in the pit of my stomach just *sensing* that something was wrong. Not the typical pain experienced by most kids at various times, Alicia's illness started as a backache. An extremely severe backache that awoke her one night and progressively got worse. Through a series of doctor's visits and medical tests to rule out a fracture to her spine, rheumatoid arthritis, and *growing pains*, we could not find out what was wrong all the while Alicia was getting progressively worse. She ailed for over a month, feeling somewhat better during the day, only to have the pain quickly return at night; becoming so unbearable, it prevented her from lying down flat. Her sleeping routine became a dose of prescription strength pain medication in the evening, sitting upright in bed on a backrest watching *Nick at Nite*. She would dose off for a short while only to be suddenly awakened by a pain that was so excruciating she would cry that no one was able to help her. She cried, I cried, and as each night passed, that sick feeling in the pit of my stomach grew stronger. Something was terribly wrong, and I nor the medical community could not figure out what it was.

TOO MUCH INFORMATION

T HERE ARE THOSE who say the Internet is more of a curse than a blessing because it can give too much information and not necessarily the correct information. Although there were those around me who tried to discourage my searches online for pediatric back pain, out of desperation and no logical answers, I soon resorted to them. Trying to figure out what was causing Alicia so much pain and how come no one could help her was making me more uneasy. The more I read, however, the more concerned I became as my research was leading me to the belief that something major was wrong with Alicia.

DR. JOHN FIGURES IT OUT

JANUARY 15, 2002, having exhausted all other options, Alicia was scheduled to go for an MRI, magnetic resonance imaging, at my friend's radiology practice. Dr. John had already done a bone scan on her lower back, the point of origin for her pain and had found nothing. After exhausting all of our other options, Dr. John decided he needed to do an MRI. He was determined to figure out exactly what was wrong. Alicia had another terrible night the evening before her test and awoke to a new complication as the mobility in her legs was now being affected. As she stumbled around the house, getting ready to go, my heart was sinking, imagining what could possibly be so wrong it was now making her fall and unable to walk? I was terrified driving to his office yet hopeful that maybe he could figure out exactly what was going on and fix it. I never let Alicia know just how frightened I really was as I made small talk and silly conversation with her. She didn't need to know my concerns, as I was sure she had enough of her own. Mommy was trying to help her out, yet so far, she was unable to. Sometimes moms can't fix everything. Medical tests are a scary thing for anyone, no less a six-year-old child. Now added to this mix was the fact that Alicia was in such horrific pain she was unable to lie on her back. She hadn't been able to lie down flat for the past few weeks. The open MRI she was to be screened on required her to lie down. This seemingly simple feat caused her such pain it broke my heart. I could not and would not cry; however, we needed to figure out what was wrong, get it fixed, and deal with our emotions later. Arriving at the office, Dr. John quickly took note of Alicia's stumbling and irregular gait and made a medical decision that he was going to concentrate his study upon her upper spine, instead of the lower spine where she felt the pain and everyone had been looking. His assurance to me that day was he was going to get to the bottom of her problem. He would find out what was wrong. While I tried to find some relief in his assurances, at that moment it was of little comfort, knowing just how much she was going through. Alicia is a borne trouper. We explained to her what needed to be done and exactly what she could expect from the test, and she went into the test, hoping that maybe somebody could help her pain go away. I watched her go into that test with uneasiness in my heart, worrying and wondering what is wrong with my baby. Twenty minutes into the test, we found our answer. Alicia had a tumor the size of an adult index finger wedged in her spinal chord severely compressing the chord itself. Dr. John quickly pulled Alicia off the MRI once he had seen and captured it on film, and the clock started ticking in a race against time. The tumor needed to be removed as soon as possible. The day was spiraling in a whirlwind of emotion, haste, and confusion. I felt like we were unlikely candidates in a movie. While I enjoy movies and the perspective that they give us the viewer, as we get a glimpse into someone else's life, this was a movie that I did not care to be in. We were in a race against a tumor that, according to Dr. John, was at risk of severing her spinal chord. A tumor that was placing so much pressure upon her spinal chord, he could not believe she was not screaming in agony. When I heard the word *tumor*, I had to ask Dr. John the inevitable question, "Did it look cancerous?" Usually tumors meant cancer. He assured me based upon the defined borders of it that it truly didn't present itself as a cancer, and at least, whatever it was, it was contained. I did find a small sense of comfort as Dr. John conferred with his associates and immediately got on the phone to speak with Alicia's pediatrician about what was unfolding. He explained to me that Alicia was going to need major back surgery, and we were off to a pediatric neurosurgeon. She would be admitted to the hospital today, and the surgery would be taking place within the next day or two. Time was of the essence, and we had to move quickly.

Waiting at the Doctor's Office

Doctors are notorious for making us wait. Schedule an appointment show up early, and inevitably you are never seen on time. While this can seem annoying for most of us, on January 17, I truly understood and appreciated why. As the severity of Alicia's condition was unfolding, the doctors now tending to her were making her their utmost priority. Phone calls, copies of films, and the *meeting of their minds*, she was the priority at that moment. I am sure there were some patients that day who were upset they had to wait a bit longer, but everyone was there helping Alicia, and at that moment, that was the only comfort I could find from such a horrible situation. We headed out from the radiologist's office straight to the pediatric neurosurgeon, films in hand while Alicia's pediatrician was on the phone assuring us that the doctor we were going to see, Dr. Mittler, was the best. Highly regarded in his field, he had been briefed about her condition and was awaiting her arrival at his office. A friendly middle-aged doctor, he quickly won over Alicia's confidence with his expertise on SpongeBob Square Pants and an employee lounge stocked with numerous snacks and drinks. Dr. Mittler was articulate and concise in his explanation of the surgery that was required for Alicia. Immediate admittance to the hospital followed by intravenous drugs of morphine to ease her pain and steroids to minimize the swelling of her spinal chord. He explained in detail how he needed to remove the bony covering around her spinal chord to gain access to the spinal column and her tumor. He would then remove the tumor, which hopefully hadn't grown into the surrounding tissue, and he would reattach those bones back to her spine with staples. While he seemed at ease with the procedure, he did it for a living, I was horrified at the whole prospect. Alicia's spine being cut open, and immediately, I began wondering if this was going to affect her walking and if it could paralyze her for life. A very real possibility but one we had no choice about, other than to pray. This was another tough predicament for a little girl who already had been through so much in her short life.

ALL ABOUT ALICIA

ALICIA HAS HAD a tough road from the day she was born. By six months of age, I had her in an early intervention program due to sensory integration difficulties. With an inability to cope with crowds, noise, touch, and even textures of food, by eight months of age, she started intense occupational therapy. We added speech therapy when her language skills didn't develop, and eventually, by age two, I had to send her off on a minibus to a self-contained nursery school that specialized in children with developmental difficulties. Alicia has always been a fighter. As a baby, while she struggled to find comfort in her own skin, she took every challenge placed before her, and while initially seemed overwhelmed, she rose to the occasion and eventually persevered. The story of her life has been about challenge and adversity. Even the simplest of tasks was met with frustration, fear, and an eventual *overload* of emotion. I learned early on how to motivate Alicia, how to minimize stress for her, and how to push her to her limits so that she could overcome some of the issues that haunted her. Now faced with the unbelievable prognosis of spinal surgery, I could only reflect upon my memories of all she had already been through and start to formulate in my mind a plan of action to get my baby through this next seemingly insurmountable hurdle.

POLLY POCKETS TO THE RESCUE

KIDS WILL BE kids, and it was what I was now counting on to get Alicia through this next step in treating her pain. Polly Pockets, miniature dolls with tiny rubber clothing and shoes was a big favorite of Alicia's. She had wanted some new sets; and now was the time I needed to pull out all stops and just bribe, bribe, bribe. I explained to her that we now knew what was causing her the terrible pain she had when they identified her tumor. I also told her, though, that the tumor needed to come out, and the only way that could happen was surgery. She was scared, as was I, but I refused to let her know just how scared I really was. So after I explained to her that she was going to be admitted to the hospital, she was going to get medicine to take the pain away, and then we would let the doctors do what they needed to do in order to make her feel better, I also suggested we needed some Polly Pockets to play with during *our* stay at the hospital. This was going to be *our* battle, and Mommy was going to there every step of the way as I was with every other issue in her young life. The premise of parental bribery seemed simple enough in theory, yet all the while, I had an overwhelming urge to cry. My philosophy with my children was and always has been, tell them the truth as they know when you are lying to them, and while I made my explanation of what was going to happen as kid friendly as possible, it was still overwhelming just the thought of what she was facing. While I reassured her that I was going to be right there with her every step of the way, this problem was something that Mommy couldn't fix by herself; we needed the help of the doctors and nurses to make everything all right. First things first, though, as we left Dr. Mittler's office, it was off to the toy store to get some toys. I carried Alicia into a local toy store since her legs were now failing her, and we needed to make our purchases quickly and efficiently while the hospital emergency room was going to be our last stop. There she was going to get the much-needed medication to stop the excruciating pain she was experiencing. Me running around a toy store with a sixty-five-pound little girl in my arms was probably a sight to be seen, but at that time, I believe I had mustered up superhuman strength just trying to get her to make her selections so we could get to the hospital.

THE EMERGENCY ROOM

EMERGENCY ROOMS AND hospitals are not fun places to be. They are usually loud, crowded places filled with confusion and commotion. I was worried that due to her sensory sensitivities, the emergency room alone could overwhelm her before we even got to them placing an intravenous needle in her hand or administering any medication. On that January 15, though, the emergency room at North Shore University Hospital in Manhasset, New York, was eerily calm and quiet. Alicia, myself, and just a few other people waiting, it seemed more like a doctor's office than a hospital, and for this, I was extremely grateful. It made it easier for me to reassure Alicia that the hospital was not a scary place, but just like a big doctor's office. I am a spiritual individual, and while at the time, I was a catechist for J. J.'s religious education class, I always looked at my spirituality as the culmination of God's master plan. His will for us as people is what I believe is our life path and the basis of all faith. The things we are presented with during our life that help or hurt us in our journey are the *signs* for lack of a better word or the directions that God leaves for us as a *road map* for our journey. Just as Hansel and Gretel left crumbs in the woods, I believe that God gives us his own crumbs to help us find our way; it is up to us, however, to know which ones to pick up and which ones to follow. We were now faced with major back surgery for Alicia, and our first sign was about to be seen. While sitting in the emergency room filling out paperwork and medical forms, it was obvious that Alicia was troubled by this entire situation. Always one to look for a silver lining, I was assuring her that this is where we had to be, that the hospital helps many people with many medical problems. This was not something that could be done in the relative comfort of a doctor's office and that there were other people there like her, needing the expertise and the facilities that only a hospital could offer. It was during this time that a cousin of mine was walking through the emergency room. A messenger sent by God in my mind, but a reassurance to Alicia at that moment that here was a relative of ours needing the care of a hospital too. My aunt was admitted due to some age-related issues, and my cousin Chris had just brought her through the emergency room where they determined her need to stay. While a chance meeting such as this one may seem irrelevant, I looked at it as a clear-cut sign that God was with us, and he was going to give us the support we needed. Alicia felt a small sense of comfort that here was someone familiar there too; we were going to be admitted, and it was going to be okay.

NEEDLES AND OTHER SCARY STUFF

ONCE ALICIA WAS in the emergency room being tended to by a physician, it was time to try and convince her that the needle they were going to put into her hand was really *not that big of a deal.* I hate IVs myself, and if there was any way I could have had them place it into my vein instead of Alicia's, I would have done it in a heartbeat, but that is a mommy dream and not how this was going to work. After much playing, reasoning, cajoling, begging, and even more bribing, the doctor was able to get the IV needle in her hand and start a mixture of steroids to reduce the swelling of her spinal chord and morphine to finally alleviate her excruciating pain. Within minutes of administering the drugs, Alicia was finally able to get some relief. Her pained tiny face suddenly looked more peaceful as the drugs took effect, and she was able to finally feel relief. It took a long time getting to this point, but at least, I had a sense that things were getting better, and since we had identified her problem, we were now able to fix it.

OTHER OBLIGATIONS

A DAY SUCH as this one, while extremely emotional and intense, also takes you out of your everyday world and literally turns everything upside down. I had two other children at home: Lauren, grade 7 at the time, and J. J., who was in grade 4. In between all of my running, testing, and consulting regarding Alicia, there were telephone calls to my parents, the ultimate grandparents, who drove to my house to watch the other children and to various people to alert everyone to the situation as it was unfolding and to clear schedules. We were going to be in the hospital for a while, and there were many people who needed to be notified of exactly what was happening. Lauren was going to do the packing for Alicia and myself as I tried to explain to her the items we needed, from toothpaste and a toothbrush to clothes, slippers, and my contact lens case. I also wanted to see Lauren and J. J. I needed to see Lauren and J. J. I needed them to visit their sister and to understand what was happening and what this meant to them. I wanted my family around me as we were about to face something terribly frightening, so my parents were going to bring them up to the hospital to visit that night.

PARENTING BY "MOI"

AS A STAY-AT-HOME mom for my children's entire lives and being the caregiver for them, my parenting technique, while some may question as being unorthodox, has been extremely consistent. I have always treated them with respect, honesty; and while the ultimate decision-making for them was mine, I did seek input from them and tried to encourage them to openly express themselves. My kids were growing up as compassionate, insightful, and helpful people who, most of my neighbors and friends would tell me, were kids that they wished their young ones would grow up to be like. As I realized now the turmoil our family was facing, I wanted to see them all and tell them what was going to happen and what I needed each of them to do. I was anxiously awaiting their arrival at the hospital to visit Alicia and myself. "You plan and God laughs" is a very old saying that gives a very accurate perspective on life. While we are all so busy scheduling, planning, and doing, we tend to get caught up in our own self-importance of the "props being more important than the play." All of my planning had now gone right out the window, as God saw our path take a major detour right in that hospital. With the arrival at the hospital of Lauren and J. J., it was up to me to put their fears at ease as to what was going on. Alicia needed surgery, but from what the doctors had all seen from her tests and films, it looked as though as everything was going to be just fine.

RELIEF

S EEING ALICIA IN her hospital bed hooked up to intravenous drips providing her with morphine to deal with her excruciating pain and steroids to calm the swelling of her spinal chord was a frightening sight for all of us; however, she finally was out of pain. Her pain had become so severe and ever increasing on a daily basis that to now see her smiling relieved face finally made us appreciate that help was finally found, and now the doctors were going to take care of the rest. We were lucky. We found out what was wrong, and it was going to be taken care of.

PREPARING FOR SURGERY

ALICIA RESTED COMFORTABLY for the next day and a half with her surgery scheduled for Thursday, January 17. The day before surgery, a pediatric oncologist visited Alicia's room to speak to me about the possibility of the tumor in Alicia's back being cancer. It was standard hospital protocol when a patient had a tumor an oncologist would meet with the family prior to surgery as an introduction. I was in no mood to hear from an oncologist, Dr. Mark, who was doing his job. He was there to meet Alicia and to speak to me. I quickly told him that, while I appreciated what he did, I did not plan on having anything to do with him. My daughter was having spinal surgery for a tumor that, from the tests, looked like nothing more than a benign growth. I had been assured that the tumor itself had self-contained borders, and most cancers are not self-contained. This was the reasoning and explanation of the surgeon, my doctor friend, and based upon research, I had done a logical deduction, and something I was praying with all my heart was the case with Alicia. My discussion with Dr. Mark that day was more of an exercise in convincing myself that it was okay rather than anything else. Although I had done much research online regarding her symptoms, it was too unsettling to even think for a second that she could possibly have cancer.

SURGERY DAY, THURSDAY, JANUARY 17

AFTER TWO NIGHTS sleeping or at least attempting rest on a pullout hospital chair next to Alicia's bed, Thursday morning could not have arrived soon enough for me. I wanted that damn tumor out of her back. I wanted Alicia on the mend, back home, and back to our routine. Six-year-old kids belonged in school, having playdates and enjoying themselves; they did not belong in a hospital having surgery. My heart was breaking as the attendants from the operating room arrived to take Alicia downstairs. I tried to remain calm, cool, and collected as I attempted small talk with Alicia. I have an annoying habit of kidding and joking around, and this was all I could muster up at this point. I did not want her to see just how scared I was as she lay there in her bed, an IV line running from her hand and a look of bewilderment on her face. I prayed to God with all my heart to please take care of my baby for me. I had wished over and over that I could have traded places with her in that bed. Make me go through surgery, spare her all of this, but all of this was a parent's unrealistic wish in an attempt to spare my child all of this pain. I was now praying that she would get through surgery just fine, her tumor would be removed successfully, and she would walk. A tumor pressing on the spinal chord like hers presented a whole other set of issues. While we were hopeful that the spinal chord would rebound back to its original form, it was being extremely compressed, and we just didn't know if there would be any permanent damage. Alicia's surgery lasted three agonizing hours. It was a difficult time as the minutes seemed like years awaiting word from the surgeon. When Dr. Mittler finally brought me and my husband into a small consultation room, he started by telling us that the surgery was a success. He was able to remove the entire tumor. It came out in a few pieces but hadn't attached itself to the spinal chord or surrounding tissue a concern for many tumors. I took a deep breath for a fleeting second, but it was quickly extinguished by his next statement. A quick pathology test indicated that the tumor itself was a "blue cell tumor." I could not believe those words as they kept on repeating in my mind, "blue cell tumor." All of my research online had educated me as to what a blue cell tumor was, and it was the worst, it was cancer. I was shocked, outraged, and sad all at the same time. How could this be happening? My baby had a life-threatening disease! Cancer happened to other people, not us. While my mind was racing at a hundred miles an hour, I tried to focus and listen to the rest of his words. I felt as though I was in a movie. Trying to see, hear, and grasp all that was going on around me but unable to focus. I was watching and hearing things that I could not possibly be a part of. Finally, I was able to comprehend what the doctor was saying. Alicia needed additional surgery to implant a Mediport in her chest; she needed further pathology to confirm exactly what type of cancer she had and the involvement of her next set of doctors who would be treating her, oncologists. All I wanted now was to see Alicia. I needed to hug and kiss her and tell her that I loved her as I now felt as though I was entering a virtual war with a deadly disease.

A TIME TO CRY

TEARS HELP CLEANSE the soul. One of those sayings I had picked up during my childhood from an older relative, along with some other *winners*, such as "Sing while you are eating and you will grow big feet" and "Swim right after eating and you will sink like a rock." This philosophy about tears, however, was proving to be true and extremely cathartic for me as I went into the ladies room to allow myself a moment of sorrow and to let my tears flow. It was a beneficial experience, those five minutes I stood over a bathroom sink in a hospital crying. I cried for Alicia, cried for my other children who now had to be told about this horrible new reality, and I cried for the seemingly unfairness of it all. Alicia had been through so much already in her six short years with her sensory issues; this was yet another obstacle in her young life. Some splashes of cold water to the face a few Kleenexes later; I was ready to go see Alicia. I needed to put my best face forward and comfort my child. As I entered the recovery room, there were a few children in curtained cordoned cubicles, attached to various tubes and monitors. It appeared to me, they were the *lucky ones*. Tonsillectomy and myringotomy, these children came in for a procedure, would go home, and get on with their lives. There was the sound of beeping, the scurry of nurses at the nurse's station and the smell of antiseptic—a true hospital smell and a smell I was going to become all too familiar with. As I entered and rounded the curtain to where the nurses directed me, I caught my first glance of Alicia. She looked so small, frail, and vulnerable. Her eyes were closed as she was sleeping, but the maze of tubes and wires all around her made me feel sick to my stomach and feel like I was going to vomit. She was so tiny lying there, and she was so sick. Next to her bed stood a familiar face, the face that I had vowed I didn't want to see or deal with. It was the oncologist Dr. Mark, who had introduced himself to me just a day before and now was a welcomed sight. He was the doctor who was going to help Alicia with her cancer care. We exchanged some small talk and quickly got into what would be taking place within the next few days. He was a professional and an expert, and he was taking charge in caring and healing my daughter. Alicia needed to recover from major back surgery. She would be evaluated by a neurologist, she would work with a physical therapist and would mend in the hospital. We needed to get her walking again, and pathology needed to determine exactly what type of cancer Alicia had. We were faced with an unimaginable future, an uncertain future, and unfortunately, for us, it was our future. How we would get through this, only time would tell. Right now, however, I needed to comfort and love my daughter. I needed to let her know that Mommy was there, and for today with her surgery complete, she was doing just fine.

HOSPITAL LIFE

T HE NEXT FEW days were a whirlwind of tests, followed by more tests. Visitors too numerous to even keep track of and sleepless nights on that pullout chair next to Alicia's bed. While I worried about Alicia, my heart was also aching for Lauren and J. J. Having been a stay-at-home mom for my children's entire lives, they were now having to deal with the fact their younger sister had cancer, I was no longer home for them due to being with Alicia, and life as they once knew it was changing. The uncertainty of what each of us was feeling was magnified even tenfold in the lives of children. While I was an adult trying to make some sense and predict the outcome of these circumstances, for my children it had to be overwhelming. Our lives would never be the same. Each day Alicia got a bit stronger, and we were soon going home. She finally was discharged on January 23. Alicia was going home.

THERE IS NO PLACE LIKE HOME . . .

THE NEXT FEW days at home were chaotic as there was an in-home physical therapist who was working with her, countless visitors, and constant telephone calls. All of it was good, very good. Alicia was home and surrounded by her sister, brother, and all of her friends. Alicia maneuvering her wheelchair around the house was also another issue we were dealing with as she quickly became adept enough to start *racing* around the house. She had visiting nurses coming to the house to check on her and just having her back in her surroundings was good, not only for her but for my other children as well. We would face what tomorrow would bring tomorrow, for now, we were just enjoying the moment.

ALICIA UPDATES

DURING THIS TIME, in an effort to be able to communicate with all of our friends and family, I started writing *Alicia Updates*. These few paragraph summaries enabled me to effectively get to everyone concerned the information about what was going on. Making twenty telephone calls a day was not something I was capable of doing, and, therefore, I got into the habit of sending out e-mails. At first, they were short and gave some basic information. Over time, these e-mails proved to be a sort of therapy for me. An opportunity to express the horror, sadness, and even joy that not only Alicia was going through but that my other children and myself were dealing with also. They were a snapshot of a day, a moment, a thought, an emotion, and countless other elements of being human. My e-mail list grew as did what I needed to say, what I felt compelled to say. People began forwarding them to their friends, and Alicia updates grew and grew. I didn't give them much thought as I wrote them. I would sit down at the computer, and the words just seemed to flow. I believe this may have been my therapy and my salvation—an opportunity to say what I was feeling, an attempt to make some sense of it all to myself while allowing others to share in my pain, grief, triumphs, and happiness. These were my personal diary of what cancer was doing to my kids, my family, my friends, and me. I dealt with cancer care in a unique way—Rene's way. I have never been a shy, wallflower, as my friends and family knew, but now cancer was going to show the rest of the world exactly how Rene would deal with this deadly disease. A bit quirky, very unorthodox, and sometimes over the edge, it was me doing what I do best—following my heart and instinct and caring for my family in a time of crisis. I have been told that my e-mails have made people laugh and even made some people cry. They are a reflection of a journey through "cancer world," a terrible place for anybody but especially for a child. The following e-mails follow Alicia through February 2002 up until August 2003. While most just give a diary of her treatment, they delve into the very social and emotional aspect of cancer care. They approach cancer treatment from my perspective and leave a recorded memoir of one child's road to recovery.

There Can Be No Happiness If the Things We Believe Are Different Than the Things We Do . . .

Subject: Alicia Update February 24, 2002
02/24/2002 8:34:14 AM Eastern Standard Time

Alicia enjoyed her winter recess week with her brothers, sister and friends. Her hair fell out this week, and she finally got her wig (which I think she looks adorable in.) She is expected at the hospital early Monday morning for admission. Since this is our 5 days of treatment, we don't expect to be released till sometime next weekend. Some of you have asked about visiting her, and the oncologist said anyone healthy is able to visit. Hopefully, we can get some type of schooling started this week.

Although I don't get to speak with each of you individually, I just wanted to say thank you to everyone for all your love and support. Alicia doesn't really know she has a life-threatening illness, and I attribute that to the normalcy we are and will try to maintain when we are at home. Lauren and J. J. are getting to do the things they normally do and we are all trying to live life as we once did. A year of treatment is a long time, and at various points during the year I will be asking for assistance from many of you. I know everyone is willing to help, and the one thing I have never been accused of is being shy! I know where you all are! LOL

Our next update will be tomorrow from the hospital. I will email you our telephone number and room number, and yes I've already put in my request for a window bed!

Love
Rene, Alicia, Lauren and J.J.

MOMMY, I DON'T WANT TO LOSE MY HAIR . . .

CANCER PATIENTS MOST of the time lose their hair. This is a side effect from the chemotherapy and/or radiation. While hair loss seems insignificant when you are faced with a life or death situation, when it is your hair you will be losing, it becomes devastating. Alicia was most upset about her hair loss. The needles, the nausea, the loss of schooltime all paled by comparison to the loss of her crowning glory, her hair. The tears that flowed from her big brown eyes were so painful not only for me but for her brother and sister as well. Baldness in a child signifies sickness, most likely cancer—a way for the world to recognize that Alicia was very sick. I, myself, while initially not devastated by it, quickly learned a valuable lesson as to what it now all meant.

Alicia had received her first bout of chemotherapy when she was admitted to have her Mediport implanted into her chest. A Mediport is a medical device that is surgically implanted into a patient's chest, just below the collarbone that is connected to the veins leading directly into one's heart. This device allows the doctors to insert a one-inch needle into it and administer all chemotherapy, medications, take blood samples, and give transfusions to the patient. This process is known as "accessing the port." To make this more comfortable for Alicia, I would administer to her Mediport area an hour before her accessing a cream of lidocaine and prilocaine called EMLA that would deaden the area so she would not feel pain on her chest. It was like Novocain for the skin. She could feel the pressure of the nurses pushing the needle in, but she could not feel the stick of the needle itself.

Within thirty-six hours of Alicia receiving her first round of chemotherapy, her hair started to fall out. It fell out in clumps, and within a few hours, her gorgeous head of hair was everywhere. We went snow tubing with some friends the day it happened, and I remember sitting in the cafeteria eating lunch. As people passed by our table, I saw the horrified look on their faces when they caught sight of Alicia's semibalding head. Chunks of hair were missing, and it was alarming to see. I saw the faces looking at Alicia, then looking at the rest of us sitting around the table, and I saw something in their eyes that would set the tone for me for our year of treatment. I wondered just what could be going through their mind. It was obvious from their glances, they knew she was sick. Were they thanking God it wasn't them? Were they just disgusted by it? Were they wondering if she was going to die? Were they feeling sorry, not only for her but for all of us sitting around that table? Were they pitying us? I love my family and friends. I love to socialize, network, entertain, and interact with people whenever I can. I am somewhat of a social butterfly. I have always believed that the interactions I have with people have helped me become who I am. I now was wondering, were my friends going to pity us? Would they too be frightened by Alicia's cancer? Would our relationships change due to what was now going to happen? If, heaven forbid, Alicia was to die from this dreadful disease, what would happen to all of us, and how we all interact with each other then?

I vowed the day we went snow tubing that I would handle Alicia's cancer and treatment the way I saw fit. While it might go against popular opinion of what was best, only I knew what was best for my child, and I was now set on making it happen.

CANCER MAKES YOU EITHER BITTER OR BETTER

A LICIA WAS A six-year-old child who deserved to be just that, a child. While her next year would be filled with continual hospital admissions, numerous tests, treatments, and appointments, she needed to be allowed to be a kid. There were some people whose advice to me was to isolate her for the next year and keep her away from everyone other than her family. Attending school would be too risky, due to a large population of children all with potential diseases that could kill her, and socializing with friends, including sleepovers, posed the same concerns. Travel or going anywhere with her could be overwhelming, potentially compromising her immune system even further, and the side effects of the chemotherapy could render her so weak and frail it could make her even sicker. Although I heard the words they were saying, I did not believe or buy any of it. I needed to let Alicia be a kid. She needed to be doing what every other kid was doing. One, because it was what she deserved, and two, heaven forbid, she was to die from her cancer; at least our memories of her would be of her living life as a six-year-old little girl, instead of a cancer patient. Cancer was going to make us all better. Better friends and better people. We would not accept anything less.

Subject: Alicia Update February 25, 2002
02/25/2002 1:09:28 PM Eastern Standard Time

We are in room 704, and yes we have a window! Alicia has started her hydration through the mediport and is doing fine. We will start with her chemotherapy later this afternoon. If all goes well, we should be discharged sometime on Saturday. (Can't you tell the mother likes going home the best? LOL)

Regards to everyone
Rene & Alicia

Subject: Alicia Update February 26, 2002
02/26/2002 4:52:41 PM Eastern Standard Time

Alicia did well with her chemotherapy today, although it is making her very tired. I came home to be with Lauren and J.J. tonight while Alicia's nanny will stay at the hospital. Unfortunately, Alicia is both sad and mad that I left, but hopefully she will get over it. She got to go to the playroom today and make sand art and she is looking forward to playing cards tonight with grandpa.

Till tomorrow
Rene & Alicia

Subject: Alicia Update February 27, 2002
02/27/2002 12:20:23 PM Eastern Standard Time

Alicia is doing well. Her night was uneventful which was a good thing. Her Aunt and Uncle visited today and they all played cards. Her one uncle affectionately known as "Uncle Fun" came and wiggled his ears for her. Today she is enjoying watching the snow from her window, and hopefully will go to the playroom.

Lauren and J. J. had a good night also. They played, we went out to dinner, and we blasted the stereo. What could be bad?

Keep warm and dry!
Rene & Alicia

RENE A. FESLER

THINGS GO PONDER . . .

M Y E-MAILS BECAME a source of information but also of inspiration. At various times, people would send me their thoughts and reflections and items that eloquently addressed life and its trials and tribulations. I kept those that meant most to me and ones I could relate to. This following e-mail made me ponder what we were going through and really think about how I would handle the upcoming year. Would I grow strong in the face of adversity and of an unknown future, or would I crumble and become a victim of it? I knew in my heart what my instinct was telling me to do, but did I have the strength to do what I felt was best? Would I be able to handle the tears, pain, and heartache that go hand in hand when your child is fighting for her life? I knew I had no choice in the matter, but I so wanted to have some control over a situation that left us all helpless. Then one of my friends forwarded to me the following e-mail, which someone had sent to her. It crystallized for me what I needed to visualize in my mind, in order to achieve the results and outcome I so wanted for us all.

Subject: Cup of Coffee?
02/28/2002 5:17:13 PM Eastern Standard Time

Something for everyone to think about
Cup of Coffee?

A young woman went to her mother and told her about her life and how things were so hard for her. She did not know how she was going to make it and wanted to give up. She was tired of fighting and struggling.

It seemed as one problem was solved, a new one arose. Her mother took her to the kitchen and filled three pots with water. She then placed each on a high flame until the pots came to a boil. In the first pot, the mother placed carrots, in the second she placed eggs and the last, ground coffee beans.

She let them sit and boil, without saying a word. In about twenty minutes she turned off the burners. She fished the carrots out and placed them in a bowl, pulled the eggs out and placed them in a bowl. The she ladled the coffee out and placed it in a bowl.

Turning to her daughter, she asked, "tell me, what you see?"

"Carrots, eggs and coffee," the daughter replied.

She brought her closer and asked her to feel the carrots. She did and noted that they were soft. She asked her to take an egg and break it. After pulling off the shell, she observed the hard-boiled egg. Finally, she asked her to sip the coffee.

The daughter smiled, as she tasted its rich aroma. The daughter then asked, "What does it mean, mother?"

Her mother explained that each of these objects had faced the same adversity—boiling water—but each reacted differently.

The carrot went in strong, hard and unrelenting. However, after being subjected to the boiling water, it softened and became weak.

The egg had been fragile. Its thin outer shell had protected its liquid interior, but after sitting through the boiling water, its inside became hardened.

The ground coffee beans were unique, however. After they were in the boiling water they had changed the water.

"Which are you?" she asked her daughter. "When adversity knocks on your door, how do you respond? Are you a carrot, an egg or coffee beans?"

Think of this: Which am I? Am I the carrot that seems strong, but with pain and adversity, do I wilt and become soft and lose my strength?

Am I the egg that starts with a malleable heart, but changes with the heat? Did I have a fluid spirit, but after death, a breakup, a financial hardship or some other trial, have I become hardened and stiff? Does my shell look the same but on the inside am I bitter and tough with a stiff spirit and a hardened heart?

Or am I like the coffee beans? The bean actually changes the hot water, the very circumstances that bring the pain. When the water gets hot, it releases the fragrance and flavor.

If you are like the bean, when things are at their worst, you get better and change the situation around you. When the hours are the darkest and trials are their greatest, do you elevate to another level?

How do you handle adversity? ARE YOU A CARROT, AN EGG, OR A COFFEE BEAN?

Subject: Alicia Update February 28, 2002
02/28/2002 10:59:19 AM Eastern Standard Time

Alicia did well last night with her nanny staying with her. Her friends visited yesterday which made her very happy. She is still scheduled to leave Saturday morning sometime.

Lauren and J.J. are doing well and will come up to visit Alicia today.

Other than that, no news is good news!

Be well
Rene & Alicia

GRANDPARENTS THE "OTHER" PARENTS . . .

A FEW YEARS back, a political book was published called *It Takes a Village* based upon an old proverb. While I will not delve into politics here, there are people who devote their lives to this, the title and the philosophy behind this book is very real and important when raising children. As a parent we do all we possibly can for our children; however, it takes more than just a mom and dad. It takes grandparents, the extended family, friends, and neighbors. It takes a village, and with Alicia's cancer, this fact was never more evident, and it was what I was counting on to get us through this harrowing ordeal.

My parents have been the anchor in my life. Their unconditional love for me, our family, and then eventually my own family helped us all immensely as they always put their children and grandchildren first. Working class people without any formal education, family was their priority and the most important aspect of their lives. However, they could help us out they did. They gave me and my ex-husband a financial head start with down payments on all our homes, and emotionally providing comfort and guidance along the way. They were always there for us. They were selfless, never selfish, and with Alicia's diagnosis, I would learn just how selfless they would be.

Alicia was never going to be by herself in the hospital. It was a scary place and she was just a baby. I promised her she would never spend a single night alone, and while I would occasionally have to leave her bedside to go buy lunch or take a shower, she was basically going to be tended to by me or a family member the entire time she was in the hospital. While my initial goal was to rotate night shifts at the hospital between my husband and myself, I quickly learned the limitations of some fathers in his inability and unwillingness to devote other than the minimal amount of time and energy to his daughter and her care. He could not deal with any of it and made it clear to me early on. With other children to tend to at home, Nanny quickly stepped into the role as surrogate parent on those nights that I needed to be home with Lauren and J. J.

Sleeping arrangements at the hospital are not ideal for a patient, let alone the caretaker of the patient. On the nights, Nanny would be rotating with me; at seventy-three years old, Nanny would sleep on the fold-down chair next to Alicia's bedside and tend to her needs: trips to the bathroom, occluded IV tubes, nausea, bone pain, fevers, and beeping pumps. In effect, Nanny gave up numerous nights of sleep to care for her granddaughter during her hour of need. Nanny and Grandpa, who was Alicia's regular food delivery person for any and all of her cravings and constant playmate and craft person, spent countless hours, days, and nights playing cards and doing crafts with her. They both gave so readily and willingly to her treatment and care; they were and are an important part of our *village* and the positive outcome we were so fortunate to have.

Subject: Alicia Update March 1, 2002
03/01/2002 10:39:41 AM Eastern Standard Time

Alicia is doing remarkably well with this round of chemotherapy. Her oncologist said not throwing up is a "good" thing with the medications she is getting. Well, Alicia is not throwing up and is eating. Her nights are good and her spirits are high. She speaks directly to all the nurses and doctors and I am basically here to occupy space (something I'm quite good at! LOL)

All is well with Alicia and she will be home on Saturday!

Regards
Rene & Alicia

Subject: Alicia Update March 2, 2002
03/02/2002 10:00:54 AM Eastern Standard Time

I am awaiting the arrival of Alicia this morning. Her father stayed at the hospital last night and it was interesting to say the least. Apparently there was a water main break on the floor above pediatrics. According to Alicia, there was a "river" of water going down the hall it was "raining" in a lot of the rooms and although it didn't rain in Alicia's room, at 1:30 am they had to move her to another room. She said she didn't get much sleep, but she did say there was so much excitement, it was fun. I don't think anyone else saw it that way! LOL

Alicia will hopefully be home now for 2 weeks (we return to clinic on Wednesday for counts). We expect tutoring to start this week, and the following week I will try to get her into school for a few hours.

The weekend before our next hospital stay the kids and I will be on our own, so I may need some assistance. I will be in touch.

Thinking of all of you!
Rene & soon to be home Alicia

Subject: Alicia Update March 4, 2002
03/04/2002 4:00:42 PM Eastern Standard Time

Today was a busy day for Alicia. We went to her Uncle John, her radiologist's office, this morning to complete the MRI that we were unable to finish in the hospital. Of course for him she was an angel and we have that test completed.

Next we went to North Shore Hospital to get the shot of Neupogen (a medication I inject her with daily after chemotherapy), since I never received Alicia's delivery. They were not able to give her the shot due to insurance issues, which this blonde doesn't get. So we spent an hour and a half at the hospital and basically goofed around with the doctors and nurses. The only good thing was I saw one of my doctors in the hallway and he reminded me I was overdue to be seen, so I'll go visit him next week.

The highlight of Alicia's day is the first day of home schooling by her first grade teacher Mrs. Caulfield. She is patiently awaiting her arrival as I type. She truly is excited about school; J.J. is trying to understand why. LOL

Until tomorrow

Be well
Rene & Alicia

Subject: Alicia Update March 6, 2002
03/06/2002

Alicia is doing well. Today we had our own field trip to Tanger Outlets to shop. (I am training her well.) She was tired, so we took her wheel chair and we didn't stay too long. (Actually we left because I ran out of money LOL).

Her home schooling is going great! Today one of her teachers is here and we have a little classroom set up in the basement. She does her homework during the day and has class when regular school ends.

Tomorrow we go to clinic to get blood counts and start with our first shot of Aranesp (the shots to help red blood cell production). Her shots of Neupogen are going well; she lets me inject her without any tears.

All is well in the Giacalone household

Hoping everyone is well!
Rene & Alicia

Subject: Alicia Update March 7, 2002
03/07/2002 9:22:13 PM Eastern Standard Time

Today was another busy day for Alicia. We went to clinic this morning to get her counts checked, and unfortunately her red count was too low. She ended up getting a blood transfusion this afternoon. We spent the entire day at the clinic, since the transfusion itself takes three hours. She was upset, they had to access her mediport and she missed her home schooling today. She is such a tough kid though, and made the best of the situation. She appears to be doing well though (I thought she didn't look too bad when we went in) and hopefully tomorrow will be a better day. The mother is tired though, since straight from arriving home from the hospital J.J. had a school function.

Alicia is looking forward to the weekend, and hopefully now her counts are on the rebound. If the weather is nice, we will be out and about.

Hoping everyone is well!
Rene & Alicia

Subject: Alicia Update March 8, 2002
03/08/2002 8:46:35 AM Eastern Standard Time

Some of you have not had the opportunity to see Alicia in awhile, so I've included two recent photos of her with her new hairdo. Her personality fits her smile, and she is doing beautifully. Whenever you might feel a little sad, just take a look at these. You'll feel better, I know I do!

Regards,
Rene

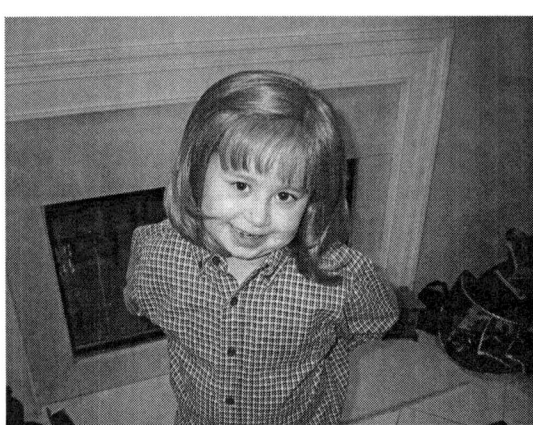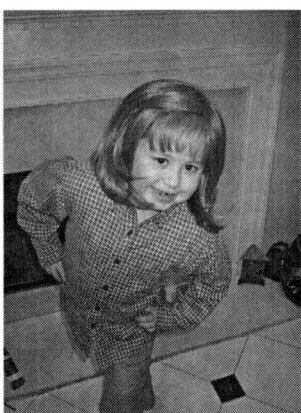

Subject: Alicia Update March 9, 2002
03/09/2002 10:01:18 PM Eastern Standard Time

Alicia is doing well today. She enjoyed the weather and played outside. This afternoon, she went with her girlfriend to get a manicure and pedicure. (What could be bad when your nails look good? LOL) she said she doesn't feel any different since her transfusion on Thursday. She said she felt good when we went in on Thursday.)

Home schooling is going great. Yesterday, her teacher stayed for 2 hours instead of the usual 1, to make up for Thursdays cancellation.

Hope everyone is doing as well as Alicia!

Regards
Rene & Alicia

LET PEOPLE HELP

A S CRAZY AND stressful as our lives had become, one lesson I learned very quickly was we were not the only ones affected by her cancer. Everyone surrounding us was impacted by her illness, and each person was learning to deal with it in their own unique way. Just as there was no life plan on how to deal with a life threatening disease when your child is sick, there was no set plan on how everyone else would deal with it as well. Our family was a work in progress, and we welcomed into our lives anyone wanting to help us. One of our dearest and oldest friends was Lauren's religious education teacher at the time, and Maureen taught me one of those valuable lessons of letting people help. Maureen wanted to do something for us. She, along with her religious education class of twelve-year-old girls, wanted to visit Alicia and bring our family dinner. With her New York City Firefighter husband, Charlie, in tow, Maureen and her class came to our home and spent an evening with us. Bringing us a fabulous home-cooked meal and dessert, the girls in her class brought Alicia presents and spent a wonderful night with our family. The interaction among the kids was priceless, and within a few minutes, I knew the importance of this visit. As Alicia—in her pajamas and robe, bald little head, and big smiling face, hugged and kissed each of the girls—I saw in each of their faces a sense of relief and acceptance with each hug Alicia gave. This was the first time any of them had seen Alicia since the start of her chemotherapy and without her hair. They had heard how sick she was, and I am sure they all walked into our house that evening with their own preconceived notion as to what Alicia looked like and how she might be feeling. I am sure they were surprised to see just how vivacious and at ease with herself Alicia was. They each got to see that Alicia was not contagious. She was still the same little girl they had all known and loved, and it was great to spend time with her. This evening of dinner, laughter, and friendship proved to be a wonderful learning process for us all. We had friends who cared and were not afraid to embrace us, and those friends got to witness that cancer may have changed what Alicia looked like, but it did not change who she was. Cancer was not going to rob us of our friends and social life. Life goes on and life is wonderful!

Subject: Alicia Update March 12, 2002
03/12/2002 4:18:31 PM Eastern Standard Time

Alicia is doing well. She is a little tired and pale, but other than that no complaints. Home schooling is going great, and she is back in the swing of doing homework.

This evening Lauren's religious education class taught by my longtime friend Maureen is making a field trip to our house. Both girls are excited since Maureen's husband Charlie, a New York City firefighter, will be accompanying them. (I have to admit, I'm just as excited, and they're bringing wine and dinner. LOL)

We go back to oncology clinic on Thursday.

Hope everyone is well!

Regards,
Rene & Alicia

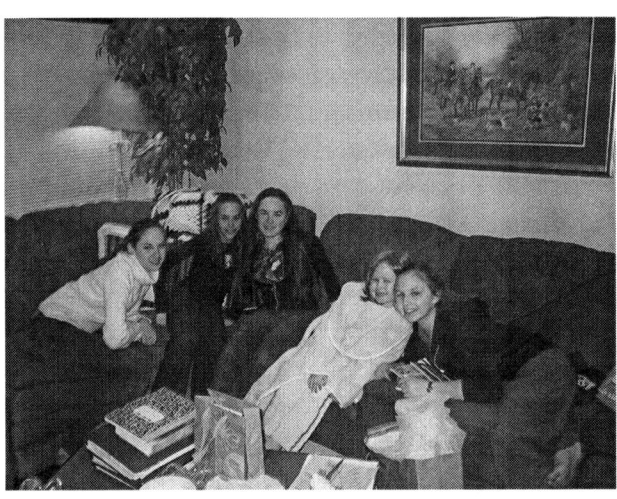

Subject: Alicia Update March 14, 2002
03/14/2002 3:01:52 PM Eastern Standard Time

We went to oncology clinic this morning and all of Alicia's numbers are good. She is feeling well and her appetite is good. After clinic, we had a field trip to a law office of some friends of ours for a visit. One of the ladies there made Alicia a beautiful rabbit doll. (When I figure out how to download from the digital camera, I'll email the picture. Cut me some slack, I'm blonde and overwhelmed!!

We are scheduled to be admitted for chemotherapy on Monday.

Hope everyone is well!
Rene & Alicia

Subject: Alicia Update March 17, 2002
03/17/2002 8:59:54 AM Eastern Standard Time

Alicia is doing fine and enjoying her weekend before her next round of chemotherapy, which starts tomorrow. Hopefully, if all goes as planned, we should only be in the hospital overnight.

I think I have found the cables to download pictures from the digital camera. I will try to figure this out today and if I do, will email some of Alicia's recent pictures.

Be well
Rene & Alicia

I wanted to forward this photo of Alicia with her handmade bunny "Louise." This was the rabbit made by Louise one of the ladies who worked at the law office we visited.

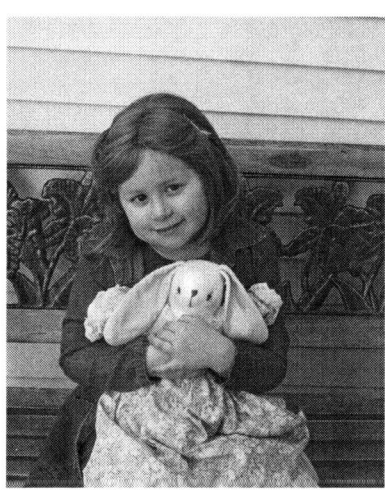

Alicia is doing well and is looking forward to a "short" hospital stay. On Friday, the oncology department of North Shore Hospital will be going to Alicia's school to speak to the teachers and students about Alicia's cancer. Alicia is looking forward to visiting with her friends.

I will let everyone know our room and telephone number tomorrow. The mother is not making a window demand, since we will only be staying overnight and we all know how "reasonable" the mother is. LOL

Be well
Rene & Alicia

Subject: Alicia Update March 18, 2002
03/18/2002 8:18:24 PM Eastern Standard Time

Alicia went into the hospital for chemotherapy today and finally got into a room (711 window, go figure) around 5:00 PM. She started her chemo this afternoon and they are promising me she will be home sometime tomorrow afternoon.

This was the first time that Alicia was agitated with the whole process. It is long, uncomfortable and boring. She is a trouper though, and after some persuasion from the mother, she settled down. As you can see from the attached photo however, Alicia and one of her oncology nurses put me in my place when I am trying to be persuasive . . . LOL. Good thing I don't take things personally!!!

Till tomorrow
Rene & Alicia

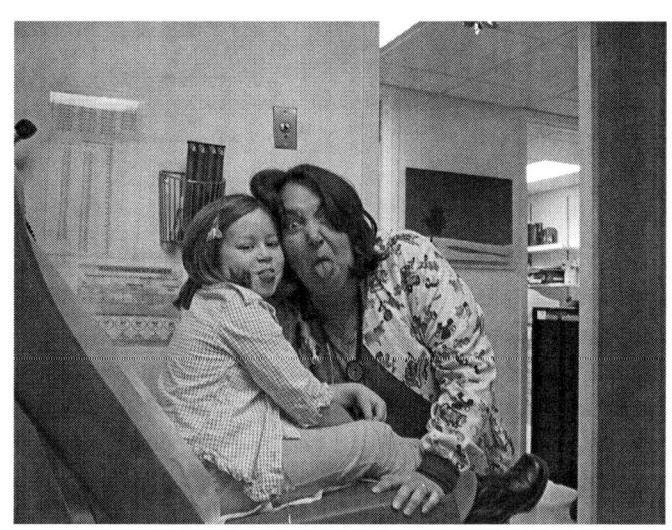

Subject: Alicia Update March 19, 2002
03/19/2002 2:14: 27 PM Eastern Standard Time

Alicia is home from the hospital. She is a little queasy, which is to be expected after chemotherapy. Her teacher is coming after school today.

All is well!
Rene & Alicia

NURSING FOR THE NON-NURSING TYPES 101

CANCER TREATMENT BECOMES more than the hospital admissions and visits to clinic for blood tests; once home from the hospital, cancer patients need medications administered daily. One part of cancer treatment I was reluctant to be involved with was injecting Alicia with medications to help her red and white counts rebound. Chemotherapy is heavy duty medications used to kill off cancer cells, which are aggressive and usually fast growing. By poisoning these cells internally when the medication is administered into the patient's blood stream, it is the goal of chemotherapy to kill off all the bad cells and to prevent them from regrowing. Radiation works by utilizing energy waves on a specific body part where cancer was present, again to kill off any microscopic cancer cells and to prevent the growth of any new cancer cells. A nurse visited our home and had to teach me how to inject Alicia with her various medications. Practicing on an orange, the consistency most like human skin, I was going to learn very quickly how to draw the medication from the vial into a syringe and then how to administer these medications to Alicia. I was probably more terrified of having to administer injections than Alicia was. I cannot tolerate blood and needles and have been known on occasion to actually pass out during my own blood tests. I would have to get over my issues and fears as now I was the one giving the shots!

THE POWER OF PEOPLE

WHILE I NEVER had a desire to be a nurse, I found myself in awe of these health care professionals who were regularly giving injections, drawing blood, and administering medications. The particular medications Alicia needed in between her chemotherapy were extremely expensive and required careful handling. Packed in ice, they needed to be kept refrigerated which made delivery of such medication critically important. The UPS man named John, who made deliveries to our home would soon become another *friend* and part of our village who made sure if we were not home to accept delivery of the medication, someone in our neighborhood would. It was during one of our first deliveries when Alicia hadn't been discharged yet from the hospital, but our delivery was on its way that the power of a friend's perseverance was exemplified. A neighbor and friend of ours named Paula was alerted to the fact that the UPS truck was going to be delivering Alicia's medication. Unfortunately, John had left a note on our front door stating that there was a package but that no one was able to accept delivery for, and therefore the package would be available at the end of the day at the UPS center around the corner from where we lived. I called Paula and let her know the circumstances, hoping that she would be able to go pick up the package from UPS. She instantly agreed to help out, and getting Alicia's medication became her mission and number one priority that day. While driving on a road near our home, she recognized our UPS driver John and flagged him down to see if he had our delivery, which he did. John pulled to the side of the road, and Paula secured Alicia's delivery of medications that day. We had a need, we asked someone to help us fulfill that need, and our friend did just that. It was a reminder to me just how important friends and family are, and if you ask people for help, they usually will. It was a team effort getting through this next year, and our team was growing.

Subject: Alicia Update March 20, 2002
03/20/2002 4:08:25 PM Eastern Standard Time

Today has been a fairly good day for Alicia. She started her Neupogen shots today (for her white count), and I had to give her a shot of Aranesp (for her red count). Unfortunately, I have to draw the Aranesp into the syringe from the vial. Of course, Alicia had loads of commentary regarding my ability to do so. We eventually did both shots with minimal amount of trauma. Alicia has been nauseous and tired today, but that is to be expected.

Unfortunately, her teacher had to cancel tutoring today. Alicia was very disappointed, since school has become a highlight for her. It seems hanging out with the mother is "boring." I always thought I was a lot of fun! LOL. Guess not.

Be well
Rene & Alicia

CANCER EDUCATION FOR KIDS

WHATEVER PROGRAM OR assistance the hospital offered to Alicia and our family, I would entertain. I had no experience within this cancer arena and therefore saw any and all resources offered us as a way to help us through this horrific time. I embraced any and all hospital staff as our lifeline and was not afraid to speak candidly about Alicia's cancer or what was going on within our family and our network. Although it was not my intention at the time, we would become a spokes family for pediatric cancer care. I looked at our fate as part of God's master plan and an opportunity to learn and grow. We all needed people, and now I was realizing just how many and how diversified a bunch of people we really did need. We were in the middle of a crisis and needed as many lifelines as we possibly could secure.

One of the programs I signed up for at the hospital was the school program allowing a team made up of an oncologist, a psychologist, and a child-life specialist to go into Alicia's school to educate both the staff and Alicia's classmates about her cancer, its effects, and what she would need when she was able to attend school. The hospital had provided to the school psychologist a letter for them to send out to the children in Alicia's class explaining that one of the children had cancer and that this program would be presented to the class on a certain date and time. Each parent had to sign a release allowing his or her child to participate in the program. There would be a presentation first and then a question and answer session. I was nervous, wondering if any of the parents would not allow his or her child to participate. How would this program be received? What questions would the children ask? How would Alicia feel knowing that this discussion was about her and her illness? I would learn from this presentation however, that the tone of Alicia's care would be defined by our attitudes and beliefs. Openness and a willingness to share our experiences was going to prove beneficial not only to us, but to everyone surrounding us. This presentation particularly the children's piece was very enlightening for me as Alicia's classmates were wide-eyed and filled with questions and comments about what she was going through. They had stories about cancer in their own families and how it affected their grandparents, aunts, or uncles. I believe it put many of their minds at ease as they had an opportunity to learn and ask questions as to what their classmate was going through. They learned that day that Alicia was still their friend, and although she was going through some pretty tough medical treatment and she looked different, she was not any different. Cancer was going to be a challenge for us but also a learning process, for everyone.

Subject: Alicia Update March 22, 2002
03/22/2002 2:43:08 PM Eastern Standard Time

Today a team from the hospital's pediatric oncology unit visited Alicia's school. First there was a presentation to the staff by one of her oncologists, Dr. Aygun along with a psychologist and a social worker. Then there was a classroom presentation to her classmates and friends. She got to spend some time in her classroom and explain what has been happening to her. We stayed at school till around 11:00 AM, when she got tired and wanted to go home.

The highlight of the visit was Alicia breaking the news to her classmates that her teacher, Mrs. Caulfield is expecting a baby. It was great day, as you can see from the attached photos. I'm down load happy; I finally learned how to work the camera! LOL

Hope everyone is doing as well as Alicia!

Rene & Alicia

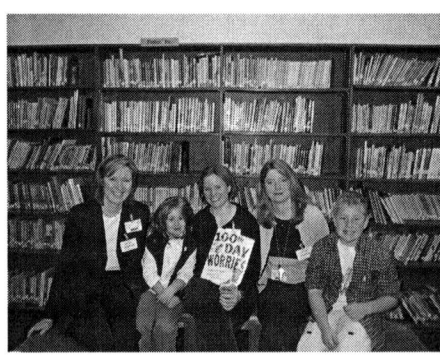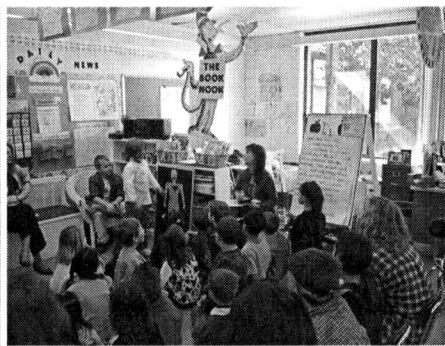

Subject: Alicia Update March 25, 2002
03/25/2002 4:54:31 PM Eastern Standard Time

We met with a radiology oncologist at Long Island Jewish hospital today, to discuss Alicia's upcoming radiation therapy. Of course Alicia was wonderful although I did get a bit cranky waiting, LOL. We expect to start radiation of her spine within the next few weeks as per her protocol.

Alicia had a good weekend. She was very very tired, and was found napping around the house a few times. We are going to clinic tomorrow for blood counts, so let's hope we don't need a transfusion.

Till tomorrow
Rene & Alicia

Subject: Alicia Update March 26, 2002
03/26/2002 1:43:11 PM Eastern Standard Time

We're back from clinic without a transfusion. HOORAY!!! Her numbers were acceptable, the white a little low. They are ordering me an additional 3 days of injections to give her, but she is doing well. She is always such a trouper.

After clinic, we do what we do best. Shop! The girls did lunch, a trip to the library, it was a good day!

We don't return to clinic until next week, and we are scheduled for next Tuesday morning for the planning and simulation for her radiation.

We now need to rest!

Be well
Rene & Alicia

Subject: Alicia Update March 30, 2002
03/30/2002 9:09:27 AM Eastern Standard Time

Alicia is doing well. She has been more tired recently, but then so is the mother LOL. We will be going to clinic on Monday to check her blood counts and to have them access her mediport. Tuesday morning she has her radiation simulation at Long Island Jewish Hospital, and will need to be given anesthesia. Alicia is more comfortable having the oncology nurses at North Shore access her mediport.

We wish everyone a good holiday!

Be well
Rene & Alicia

Subject: Alicia Update April 1, 2002
04/01/2002 9:08:32 PM Eastern Standard Time

We went to clinic today and had Alicia's mediport accessed for tomorrow's procedure at LIJ. We have to be at the hospital at 7:30 AM for anesthesia. Hopefully, the simulation should only take about an hour, but then we will have to wait for Alicia to fully recover from the sedative.

She is scheduled to start her radiation on May 2 at LIJ and will go for 25 sessions. Since we will have a conflict when we are admitted at North Shore for chemotherapy, the hospital will provide transportation via ambulance. Alicia's excited about the ride in the ambulance, she's six!

Hope everyone is well and had a wonderful holiday!

Rene & Alicia

Subject: Alicia Update April 2, 2002
04/02/2002 11:48:30 AM Eastern Standard Time

We are back from Alicia's simulation and she did great! She didn't even need anesthesia. She was able to lie perfectly still for a CAT scan, the body casting and the tattooing. We accessed her mediport for nothing, but that is OK.

Attached is a photo(s). Don't email me that you couldn't open the pictures.

Have a good day!
Rene & Alicia

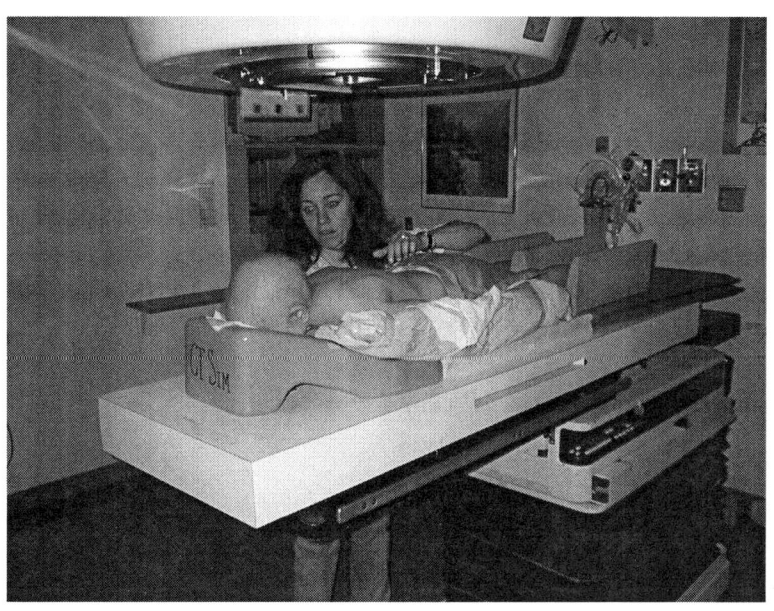

Subject: Alicia Update April 7, 2002
04/07/2002 9:36:09 AM Eastern Standard Time

Alicia enjoyed this past week with all her friends. She is feeling well, other than being tired. We are preparing for her admittance to the hospital tomorrow, if her counts are okay, for her 5 day round of chemotherapy. This is a tough stay because it is for 6 days, and the weather is getting nicer. She would rather be home playing with her friends, me too! However, we remain positive and focused and she is looking forward to some of her friends visiting her at the hospital this week and yes, the mother has already put in the request for the window! LOL

Be well
Rene & Alicia

Subject: Alicia Update April 8, 2002
04/08/2002 4:12:26 PM Eastern Daylight Time

We are admitted to room 717 door (the mother has already requested to be moved once a window bed becomes available.) Unfortunately, this has been one of the toughest admittances to date, since they couldn't get her mediport to operate properly and had to access it twice. I don't think I would be too happy with people shoving needles into my chest. Alicia cried a lot today, it has been tough for her and it has broken my heart.

She is currently getting her chemotherapy drip as I write.

Be well
Rene & Alicia

Subject: Alicia Update April 9, 2002

Alicia had to have her mediport accessed for the third time today. There was a problem with its ability to flow and therefore to accept the chemotherapy. Hopefully, this will be the last access for this visit.

Her night was a little restless with mediport problems, so the mother is a little cranky. I get to go home this evening and get some rest.

Let's hope the rest of this admittance is uneventful.

Wishing everyone well
Rene & Alicia

Subject: Alicia Update April 10, 2002
04/10/2002 10:15:04 PM Eastern Daylight Time

Just a quick note; Alicia was still having some difficulties with her mediport. She had a busy day though with lots of visitors. Unfortunately, the tutor who was supposed to start this week at the hospital has quit, therefore there will be no schooling while she's in the hospital. They are doing lots of construction in the hospital, so they test the fire alarm at least 20 times a day (Oh Lord) and there is a problem with the mother's computer. This is like a Murphy's Law stay.

Hope everyone else is doing better than us! LOL

Rene & Alicia

"THIS IS THE OPERATOR CALLING"

EVERY ADMITTANCE, ALICIA would be assigned a new telephone number. With our very first stay in January, we determined that the hospital telephone system was limited in the numbers you could dial. We lived in a different county which had a different area code and therefore we were *blocked* from making calls to our home. The hospital operators were wonderful and attentive to our dilemma and had our area code added to the system in order for us to be able to phone home. Cell phone use was banned; therefore, we needed to use the landline. With Alicia's initial admittances, the telephone calls coming to her were continual and numerous. One of the operators named Denise quickly learned there was a six-year-old on the pediatric floor, and she was continually being admitted. One day, Denise called to let us know that the technical issues we had with the telephone were fixed, and I was not in the room when this call came in. Alicia had answered the telephone and proceeded to have a lengthy conversation with her. The two struck up an instant rapport, and Denise told Alicia she could call her whenever she wanted to chat. Alicia believed her and took her up on her word. Whenever we were admitted, Alicia would call Denise to let her know she was back in the hospital, and if she wasn't in, she left a message for her. Denise would call her back and even came to visit Alicia during her lunch hour. Throughout treatment, Alicia became comfortable knowing there would be a familiar voice on the other end of the phone. While other kids were in school learning, out at recess, and doing art projects, Alicia found a *friend* in a lady who directed calls all day. Denise called often and, willingly, and Alicia loved it. She was another blessing in our lives and another reminder that support and understanding was everywhere. It was up to us, however, to reach out for it. Alicia had absolutely no problem doing this.

Subject: Hospital telephone news!
04/11/2002 7:44:14 PM Eastern Daylight Time

If anyone has been trying to contact us at the hospital, it only came to my attention this afternoon that our number is temperamental. Some people can call it direct, others cannot (it rings and rings forever, just not in Alicia's room.) If you need to contact us and can't, call the main hospital number and ask for Alicia. The operators know who she is. LOL

This is turning into the stay from Hell! Only kidding, just my warped sense of humor!

Things were actually good today. I overtook a hospital computer to get this email out.

Be Well
Rene & Alicia

Subject: Alicia Update April 13, 2002
04/13/2002 3:23:09 PM Eastern Daylight Time

Just a note to let you know Alicia came home around noon today. She is out side selling lemonade with her friends and enjoying the beautiful weather. Let's just say that this was not our "best" admittance, but it always could be worse. It is all in your perspective. We just need to count our blessings!

We go to clinic on Wednesday

Be well
Rene & Alicia

Subject: Alicia Update April 17, 2002
04/17/2002 1:26:13 PM Eastern Daylight Time

Alicia went to clinic this morning. Her red count was 8.1 (the minimum they will accept is 8). She could have gotten a transfusion today, but the mother wanted to get out and enjoy the beautiful Florida-like weather. For my Floridian friends, it is hotter here than in Naples. I love it!!!)

I need to watch Alicia the next few days to see if she is tiring more easily and monitor her heart rate. If it appears he numbers are going lower, we will need to go in for a transfusion immediately. At a minimum though, she will be back at clinic on Monday.

Hope everyone is well!
Rene & Alicia

Subject: Positive Thinking
04/22/2002 8:16:44 AM Eastern Daylight Time

Positive Thinking

Someone once had a very special teacher in high school many years ago whose husband died suddenly of a heart attack. About a week after his death, she shared some of her insight with a classroom of students.

As the late afternoon sun came streaming in through the classroom windows and the class was nearly over, she moved a few things aside on the edge of her desk and sat down there. With a gentle look of reflection on her face, she paused and said, "Before class is over, I would like to share with all of you, a thought that is unrelated to class, but which I feel is very important."

Each of us is put here on earth to learn, share, love appreciate and give of ourselves. None of us knows when this fantastic experience will end. It can be taken away at any moment. Perhaps this is God's way of telling us that we must make the most out of every single day.

Her eyes, beginning to water, she went on, "So I would like you all to make me a promise. From now on, on your way to school, or on your way home, find something beautiful to notice. It doesn't have to be something you see. It could be a scent—perhaps of freshly baked bread wafting out of someone's house, or it could be the sound of a breeze slightly rustling the leaves in the trees, or the way the morning light catches one autumn leaf as it falls gently to the ground. Please look at these things and cherish them, for although it may sound trite to some, these things are the 'stuff' of life. The little things are put here on earth to enjoy. The things we often take for granted. We must make it important to notice them, for at any time, it can all be taken away."

The class went completely quiet. We all picked up our books and filed out of the room silently. That afternoon, I noticed more things on my way home from school than I had the whole semester.

Every once in awhile, I think of that teacher and remember what an impression she made on all of us and I try to appreciate all of those things that sometimes we all overlook. Take notice of something special you see on your lunch hour today. Go barefoot. Walk on the beach at sunset. Stop off on the way home tonight and get a double dip ice cream cone. Life is not measured by the number of breaths we take, but by the moments that take our breath away. For as we get older, it is not the things we did we often regret, but the things we didn't do.

Stop a minute and thank God for all the beautiful things He's given us.

You will immediately feel a sense of comfort.

COMFORTABLE IN YOUR OWN SKIN

I T WAS TOUGH for Alicia as it is with any cancer patient because you really never feel good. All the medications, testing, and radiation—all make you feel sick, add to that a major change in appearance, and there is a lot to be upset about. With Alicia still trying to get comfortable with the loss of her hair, it was something I had a tough time talking to her about since I had never lost my hair. My words would mean nothing since I had not experienced this. One day, after a visit to clinic, we bumped into a neighborhood friend of mine in McDonald's. Noreen had been battling cancer since her daughter, who was Lauren's age, was eighteen months old. She would be declared disease free for a few years, and then her cancer would return. She had recently been diagnosed with lung cancer, and I had not seen her since. On this particular day, Noreen was in McDonald's and came over to speak with me but more importantly Alicia. She was wonderful as she told Alicia she heard she had cancer and that she had cancer too. She told her how brave she was and that she knew she would do well because she was tough, much tougher than cancer. She then removed her wig and showed Alicia her bald head. Alicia was in awe as Noreen explained to Alicia that was probably one of the best parts of cancer because she didn't have to deal with haircuts, washing, styling, and all the other responsibilities of having hair. I know that both Alicia and I would rather have had her not be sick and have a head of hair to tend to; however, that day in the middle of a fast-food restaurant, Alicia got to relate to someone who was "walking the same walk." That chance meeting was a comfort to Alicia and a lesson to me that while I could try and handle all issues relating to her cancer, there were some things that even I could not relate to or help her feel better about since I had not experience what she had. There were, however, friends like Noreen who could.

Subject: Alicia Update April 22, 2002
04/22/2002 2:04:09 PM Eastern Daylight Time

I am happy to report that Alicia made her numbers today and didn't need a transfusion. We were out of the hospital in about an hour's time (a record). Alicia wanted McDonald's, not one of my personal favorites, but she is the boss. Nanny and Grandpa met us. We met a friend of mine Noreen, who has battled breast cancer for many years and is now battling lung cancer. She and Alicia joked about wigs and being bald. It was quite a moment there in the middle of a fast food restaurant. It was a good day.

We don't need to go back until she is admitted next Monday.

Be well
Rene & Alicia

Subject: Life's Perspective
04/25/2002 3:57:48 PM Eastern Daylight Time

Someone sent me this email. I believe it was written by an author, Rabbi Krohn, and I love its message.

This will give you chills but puts life into perspective!

At a fundraising dinner for a school that serves learning disabled children, the father of one of the school's students delivered a speech that would never be forgotten by all who attended.

After extolling the school and its dedicated staff, he offered a question.

"Everything God does is done with perfection. Yet my son, Shay, cannot learn things as other children do. He cannot understand things as other children do. Where is God's plan reflected in my son?"

The audience was stilled by the query.

The father continued, "I believe that when God brings a child like Shay into the world, an opportunity to realize the Divine Plan presents itself and it comes in the way people treat that child."

Then he told the following story.

Shay and his father had walked past a park where some boys Shay knew were playing baseball. Shay asked, "Do you think they will let me play?"

Shay's father knew that most boys would not want him on their team. But the father also understood that if his son were allowed to play it would give him a much needed sense of belonging.

Shay's father approached one of the boys on the field and asked if Shay could play. The boy looked around for guidance from his teammates. Getting none, he took matters into his own hands and said, "We are losing by six runs, and the game is in the eighth inning. I guess he can be on our team and I'll try and put him up at bat in the ninth inning."

In the bottom of the eighth inning, Shay's team scored a few runs but was still behind by three. At the top of the ninth inning Shay put on a glove and played in the outfield. Although no hits came his way, he was obviously ecstatic just to be on the field, grinning from ear to ear as he father waved to him from the stands.

In the bottom of the ninth inning, Shay's team scored again.

Now with two outs and bases loaded, the potential winning run was on base. Shay was scheduled to be the next at bat. Would the team actually let Shay bat at this juncture and give away their chance to win the game?

Surprisingly, Shay was given the bat. Everyone knew that a hit was all but impossible because Shay didn't even know how to hold the bat properly, much less connect with the ball. However, as Shay stepped up to the plate, the pitcher moved a few steps to lob the ball in softly so Shay could at least be able to make contact. The first pitch came and Shay swung clumsily and missed. The pitcher again took a few steps forward to toss the ball softly toward Shay. As the pitch came in, Shay swung at the ball and hit a slow ground ball to the pitcher. The pitcher picked up the soft grounder and could easily have thrown the ball to the first baseman. Shay would have been out and that would have been the ended the game.

Instead, the pitcher took the ball and threw it on a high arc to the right field, far beyond the reach of the first baseman. Everyone started yelling, "Shay, run to first, run to first!"

Never in his life had Shay ever made it to first base. He scampered down the baseline, wide eyed and startled. Everyone yelled, "Run to second, run to second!" By the time Shay was rounding first base, the right fielder had the ball. He could have thrown the ball to the second baseman for a tag, but the right fielder understood what the pitcher's intentions had been, so he threw the ball high and far over the third baseman's head.

Shay ran towards second base as the runners ahead of him deliriously circled the bases towards home.

As Shay reached second base the opposing shortstop ran to him, turned him in the direction of third base and shouted, "Run to third!"

As Shay rounded third, the boys from both teams were screaming, "Shay! Run home!"

"That day," said the father softly with tears now rolling down his face, "the boys from both teams helped bring a piece of the Divine Plan into the world."

A footnote to this story, we all send thousands of jokes through email without a second thought, but when it comes to sending messages regarding life choices, people think twice about sharing.

The crude, vulgar and sometimes obscene pass freely through cyberspace, but public discussion of decency is too often suppressed in school and the work place. If you are thinking about forwarding this message, you are probably thinking about which people on your address list aren't appropriate ones to receive this type of message.

The person who sent this to you believes that we can all make a difference. We all have thousands of opportunities a day to help realize God's plan.

So many seemingly trivial interactions between two people present us with a choice:

Do we pass along a spark of the Divine? Or do we pass up that opportunity, and leave the world a bit colder place in the process?

You have two choices now;

1. Delete this
2. Forward it to the people you care about.

You know the choice I made.

This was Alicia from birth to age five. At the time I didn't truly comprehend all the heartache and difficulties she and our family was facing. Now at age six we are faced with a different set of circumstances. There are days things just seem insurmountable and it is very easy to become overwhelmed. However, I truly believe there is a reason Alicia is going through what she is. She is an example to everyone who comes in contact with her that courage comes in all shapes and sizes.

To everyone who has been so kind and helpful to us, a heartfelt thank you. No matter how insignificant you think your gesture may be, it is not. Every bit of assistance is cherished and appreciated more than you will ever know. If I could turn back the hands of time I would. Instead we try to make the best of each and everyday and count our blessings. Life can change in a heartbeat, so never take anything or anyone for granted!

Be well
Rene & Alicia

Subject: Alicia Update April 26, 2002
04/26/2002 3:32:48 PM Eastern Daylight Time

Want to joyfully report Alicia went to school today! I dropped her off at 9:00 AM and she lasted the whole day, when I picked her up at 3:00 PM. She was very excited to sit at her desk and see her friends.

We are looking forward to a good weekend with lots of activities, before our admittance on Monday morning. This is only a 2 day cycle, so we will be home Tuesday afternoon. Radiation on her spine starts Thursday morning.

Be well
Rene & Alicia

Subject: Alicia Update April 29, 2002
04/29/2002 2:51:07 PM Eastern Daylight Time

We are admitted in room 722 and we didn't get the window. The blonde is losing her touch LOL.

RENE A. FESLER

I hate to admit it, but coming in is getting more difficult each time. I cannot imagine what cycle 17 will be like. Remembering how difficult it was to access her port her last visit, Alicia does not want anyone going near her mediport and just cries to go home. She doesn't want to have cancer and just wants to be like other kids. It is heartbreaking to watch, but as I have told Alicia I don't want to get any older, some things are just beyond our control. The good thing is however, once she is in her room, she quickly returns to her mayoral role and starts ruling the floor. She has learned well! LOL.

She needed an echocardiogram today, so we have yet to start her chemotherapy. I have let them know that we need to be home by 6 PM tomorrow to prepare our snacks for the 7 PM puck drop of the Islanders vs. Toronto!

Hope everyone is well!
Rene & Alicia

Subject: Alicia Update April 30, 2002
04/30/2002 3:48:24 PM Eastern Daylight Time

I am happy to report, Alicia is home. She finished her chemotherapy around noon and we were discharged by 2:00 PM. Unfortunately, de-accessing her mediport was difficult. I know I would be upset having people put in than take out one inch needles from my chest also.

One of her oncology nurses Jill, an Islander fanatic, brought in some Islander stuff to decorate for tonight's game. Alicia worked all morning on some of her own decorations and after baking a cake for tonight's festivities, hopefully this afternoon will soon be long forgotten.

We both need to rest since you really don't get to sleep in the hospital! LOL

Be Well
Rene & Alicia

Subject: Alicia Update May 2, 2002
05/02/2002 5:09:22 PM Eastern Daylight Time

Murphy's Law seems to be our new motto. We went for Alicia's radiation port verification, which basically makes sure everything matches as a set up for her radiation.

Unfortunately, Alicia has lost a little weight and is no longer bloated and therefore the body cast they made for her is now too big. They tried to re-cast another one, but they were still having a hard time getting a tight fit. We had to go back after lunch for them to make another type of cast that Alicia lays in. They needed to make some special tattoos on her back as marking points for the radiation and hopefully she is now set. All of this additional re-casting however, has put us back a day. We will be going in tomorrow for port verification and the actual radiation will start on Monday.

Alicia is doing just fine, as always although I am now stressing to the point that my jaw is locking. (Some think this is not necessarily a bad thing LOL). I might have to be quiet for a little while, but I can guarantee it won't be for long though! LOL

Hope everyone is doing just fine!
Rene & Alicia

Subject: Alicia Update May 3, 2002
05/03/2002 4:52:05 PM Eastern Daylight Time

Alicia did well today with her port simulation. This is basically a series of x-rays with her in a body cast to check the entry points and paths of radiation. She actually fell asleep during this procedure.

She missed school yesterday and today she was just too tired. I have to admit all this running is making me more tired also. She is experiencing a sore throat and sniffles; let's just hope its allergies.

Monday is her first day of radiation.

Have a great weekend!
Rene & Alicia

Subject: Alicia Update May 6, 2002
05/06/2002 5:11:21 PM Eastern Daylight Time

We didn't start radiation today! Her radiation oncologist was not happy with her x-rays they took on Friday. Her upper spine alignment was off by 4 millimeters, which is unacceptable. We need to start from scratch. Wednesday at 1:30 she will have a CAT scan and they will make a new type of body cast. Of course this is now going to conflict with her chemotherapy cycle, but what can you do? As usual, Alicia is a trouper! I am not to sure about me, but Alicia is hanging tough LOL.

We are due at clinic tomorrow for counts. Unfortunately, Alicia has had an on again off again fever again. I will be packing expecting to be admitted tomorrow. If we aren't admitted, it's a bonus!

Hope all is well in the rest of the world! LOL
Rene & Alicia

Subject: Alicia Update May 7, 2002
05/07/2002 2:31:04 PM Eastern Daylight Time

We got out of clinic today without a transfusion and without a fever (Tylenol and ice water works wonders LOL). Alicia's red count barely made it, but the mother insisted we were not spending such a beautiful day in the hospital. We have places to go and people to meet! We will have to go back on Friday, and if her numbers haven't rebounded enough, she will need a transfusion. They have now put her on iron supplements, so between that and the shots of Aranesp, hopefully she will do fine.

Got to go!

Be well
Rene & Alicia

Subject: Alicia Update May 9, 2002
05/09/2002 3:27:21 PM Eastern Daylight Time

I think they finally got the body cast right after 4 times! God bless Alicia's patience through all of this. I don't think I would have been as cooperative. Unfortunately, she has to lay face down with her hands on her side, inside a body mold. The good news is, for her cooperation and sunny disposition; she is earning "rewards." Hey presents motivate me too LOL. My motto, "whatever works?"

We don't go back for port simulation until next Tuesday, thank goodness for this little breather. However, we do have to return to clinic tomorrow for a possible transfusion.

As long as we are done in time for tomorrow nights METS game at Shea Stadium. I told you we have places to go and things to do!

Hope everyone is smiling!
Rene & Alicia

Subject: Alicia Update May 10, 2002
05/10/2002 12:05:45 PM Eastern Daylight Time

We got out of clinic today without a transfusion! Although her red count was not particularly high, it was high enough to squeak by. Both mother and child are exhausted from this extremely long and stressful week. We will be resting for tonight's METS game!

Hope everyone has a wonderful weekend.

Happy Mother's Day!
Rene & Alicia

I AM TIRED AND DON'T WANT
TO DO THIS ANYMORE . . .

CANCER TREATMENT IS intense. The hospital stays, clinic visits, radiation, and transfusions—it got more difficult each and every time I had to bring Alicia in. It broke my heart when she would cry and voice her opinion that she didn't want to do it anymore. She just wanted to be like her friends—go to school, play soccer, and have sleepovers. I felt her pain, but it was now that I had to pull my parental rank and set her straight. Her having cancer was unfair, we knew that; treatment was intense and sometimes painful; we knew that too; however, fighting her cancer was the most important thing in our lives at that moment, and we were going to battle it in one of two ways. She could go willingly and make the best of it or I would physically carry her in, over my shoulder if need be, but she had no option for treatment. I was her mother, and I was going to fight for her life with all of my might, her might, and the might of everyone around us. Her choice was not whether or not she was going to be treated; her choice was how she would go to that treatment, the easy way or the hard way.

Subject: Alicia Update May 13, 2002
05/13/2002 4:18:06 PM Eastern Daylight Time

Alicia went to school today! She was excited about going and stayed until the end when she finally got tired and needed to be picked up. I am planning on sending her Wednesday and Friday if she is able, since these days don't conflict with clinic and radiation. Next week we are going in for her 5 day chemo cycle, so let her enjoy some time in school.

We are hanging in, although it is getting tougher for Alicia. She has voiced her opinion that she doesn't want to do chemotherapy or radiation anymore. I have explained to her that there are things she has control over, and things she doesn't. Going to school for her is an option, refusing treatment is not! I have to admit, she is giving me a run for my money and they say the fruit doesn't fall far from the tree. With a mother like moi no wonder the child is so headstrong LOL. The mother will prevail however, since I don't like losing!

Lauren and J.J. are doing well. They are such great kids. Things WILL be fine though, because we wont settle on anything less!

Be well
Rene & Alicia

LIFE'S LITTLE TREASURES

IN AN ATTEMPT to maintain a *normal* life for all of my kids, I tried as hard as I could to do the things that we would do if Alicia hadn't been sick. J. J.'s fourth grade class had an ongoing project that spring of hatching eggs. The eggs sat under heat lamps, and each day, J. J. would joyfully report, as one by one the eggs hatched. Students in the class had the opportunity to take the baby chicks home for an evening. Of course, J. J. wanted the same chance, as did his classmates, and Alicia too was thrilled with the prospect of bringing baby chicks home. Alicia's oncologist was not happy after I informed him *after* the fact that I had baby chicks in the house (little petri dishes of disease), but the joy they brought to J. J. and Alicia (Lauren wasn't as thrilled) was priceless. With careful hand washing and the cage delegated to the family room, the baby chicks were adorable and lively, and the kids were thrilled with them. Life goes on, and I wanted us all to be part of it, we had to be part of it. Chicks and all, life and laughter was for the living, and that's exactly where we needed to be.

Subject: Alicia Update May 16, 2002
05/16/2002 1:13:05 PM Eastern Daylight Time

Alicia did radiation today for the first time and without a problem! Straight from the hospital we went to Alicia and J.J.'s school to pick up some baby chicks for the evening. J.J.'s class has hatched some eggs and all the children have the opportunity to bring one home. Of course we couldn't miss out on this chance, so we ended up with two chicks, one for Alicia and one for J.J. Cancer I can handle, I am not too sure about livestock!

Alicia plans on attending school again tomorrow, since we have an evening radiation appointment. The mother is not going to know what to do with her free time!

Enjoy your day!
Rene & Alicia

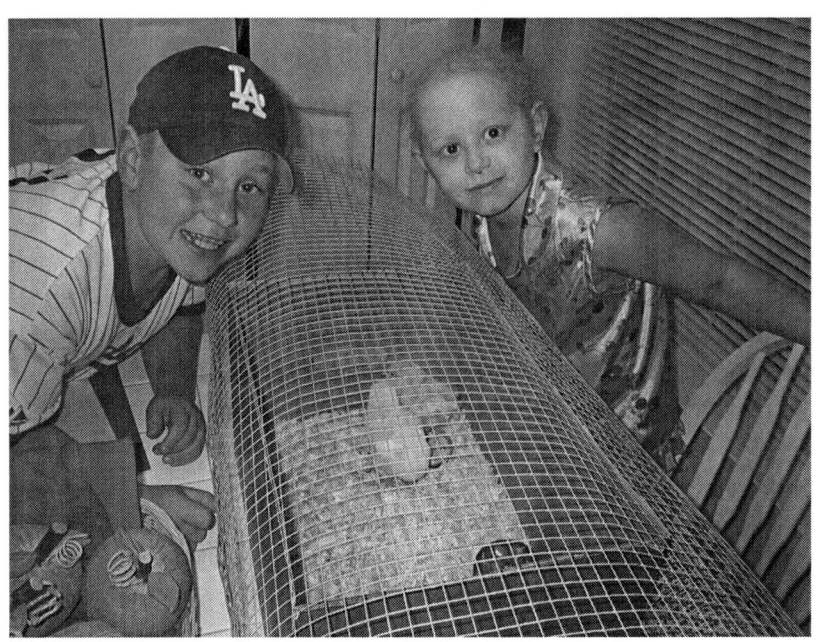

Subject: Alicia Update May 19, 2002
05/19/2002 10:16:48 PM Eastern Daylight Time

Alicia has been very busy the past few days. Friday she spent the whole day in school and had a good session of radiation. Saturday she had her friends communion party and Sunday she went with Lauren, J.J. and some friends to the NYPD vs. NYFD football game at Giants stadium.

We will do radiation tomorrow at LIJ first, and then go straight to North Shore for admittance and chemotherapy. This is the six day stay, and Alicia is not that happy to be away from home for that long. (The mother isn't either). The good news is, Alicia gets to ride in an ambulance.

I will not be bringing my computer to the hospital since we will be shuffling back and forth between two hospitals and with my luck I will forget it somewhere. I will "borrow" a hospital computer to send out our telephone number.

Hope everyone is well!
Rene & Alicia

Subject: Alicia Update May 20, 2002
05/20/2002 1:37:06 PM Eastern Daylight Time

Alicia is admitted, room 708 and yes we got a window. This is the first room we were admitted to for Alicia's back surgery. The mother brought the computer; Alicia asked how we could play pinball if we didn't bring the laptop. Her mediport was accessed with minimal tears, and radiation went well this morning.

Unfortunately, J.J. had to be picked up from school early. He gets a stomach ache every time Alicia and I are admitted. Someone does miss me when I'm not home! LOL

Hope everyone is well
Rene & Alicia

Subject: Alicia Update May 21, 2002
05/21/2002 09:21:27 PM Eastern Daylight Time

We were transported today to LIJ by ambulance. The entire roundtrip was about an hour, including treatment. Alicia has been a little more tired and quieter this stay. The whole pediatric ward is quieter since as of today there was only sixteen kids on the whole floor. (We like having our own room. The staff hangs out with us during their breaks!)

I am home for the next 2 nights to spend time with Lauren and J.J. Life is good when you get a chance to sleep! LOL.

Hope all is well.
Rene & Alicia

Subject: Alicia Update May 22, 2002
05/22/2002 06:56:19 PM Eastern Daylight Time

Alicia did well again today with radiation, even though she is a little down. We have the ambulance transportation down to a science, and roundtrip took about an hour. Alicia needed some additional x-rays today due to the fact with chemotherapy they keep her so well hydrated; she has put on about 2 pounds since Monday. They wanted to make sure the tattoos on her back lined up properly. The mother's motto, "never too cautious."

When we returned from radiation, Alicia started her chemotherapy. Unfortunately, she will be getting a transfusion this evening since her red count is only 8.5 and when you are getting radiation you need a minimum of 10.

Her pediatric neurosurgeon popped in to see her this morning and she was able to stump him with a "Sponge Bob Square Pants" question. (He has a 7 year old at home).

The afternoon the room turned into a nail salon with one of the nursing assistants, Wendy doing everyone's nails including Alicia and even nanny.

The mother lay in Alicia's bed all afternoon, hey she was sitting in my chair and then I returned home to attend Lauren's band concert this evening.

Tomorrow we are planning on breaking out of the pediatric ward in the afternoon to enjoy some sunshine. The staff made the mistake of giving me the code to the back door, so now we can move in and out of the ward undetected! I just love breaking the rules!

Be well
Rene & Alicia

Subject: Alicia Update May 24, 2002
05/24/2002 9:41:43 AM Eastern Daylight Time

Thank goodness it is Friday! The week has been going relatively well. Unfortunately, the combination of radiation and chemotherapy has made Alicia throw up. For those of you who remember, the mother is quite good at catching vomit! We are lucky that throwing up doesn't faze her.

Yesterday we had a little difficulty with hydration after radiation. Between drinking and intravenous Alicia had over 30 ounces of fluid. She only gave back about 6 ounces so we had to play a chug a lug game to force more fluids through her. We finally got her hydrated enough to start chemotherapy at 5:30 PM, but because of all of this, we didn't get to go outside. We did however walk out of radiation oncology, to wait for our return ambulance outside. The staff said, "you're not supposed to do that!" My response, "six year olds are not supposed to get cancer either, see you tomorrow!"

RENE A. FESLER

We have already started our drinking for the day, so we can hopefully get chemotherapy started earlier. The earlier it starts today, the earlier the discharge tomorrow; Alicia has a luau, hot tub, sleepover party tomorrow evening. She has a better social life than me!

Nanny will be staying the night with Alicia while the mother will be running between soccer and baseball then hopefully hot tub and some rest!

Hope everyone has a wonderful holiday weekend!
Rene & Alicia

Subject: Alicia Update May 29, 2002
05/29/2002 1:04:48 PM Eastern Daylight Time

Alicia had a wonderful weekend with parties and playing with her friends. Due to the radiation and chemotherapy combination, she has been getting "sick" more often, but not enough to slow her down.

We went to clinic today for a numbers check and were expecting a transfusion due to the need for a higher red count with radiation. She was lucky though, her counts were good and no transfusion was needed. From North Shore we went to LIJ for radiation and she was all done by noon. Alicia went to her nanny and grandpa's for the rest of the day and a sleepover. She will do radiation with my parents tomorrow since I am going on a field trip with J.J. I'm not quite sure where we are going, but I am going!

Since Alicia is gone, it is just Lauren, J.J. and I. Sounds like a good night to be a couch potato and watch some ice hockey!

Hope everyone is doing well.
Rene & Alicia

Subject: Alicia Update June 2
06/02/2002 10:08:21 PM Eastern Daylight Time

Alicia had another wonderful weekend packed with parties and playing with friends. She tried to go to school on Friday, but the radiation is making her tired and she wasn't able to go. (The radiation is making the mother tired.) She still has about 15 more radiation sessions, and we are finding that is it causing more frequent vomiting.

We will go to clinic on Wednesday and hopefully NOT need a transfusion. Cancer sure keeps you busy! We are staying positive and just trying to live each day to the fullest.

Hope you are all doing the same!
Rene & Alicia

Subject: Alicia Update June 4
06/04/2002 1:52:55 PM Eastern Standard Time

We are plugging along with radiation almost half way done. One of the difficulties we face is the logistics of radiation on a clinic day. If Alicia needs a transfusion, her port needs to be accessed and then her blood sent for a type and cross. This alone could take a few hours, and the transfusion itself is three hours. The mother, always looking to minimize our time at the hospital, decided to go to clinic today after radiation to check on her numbers. If she needed a transfusion, we would access her today, get the sample send and then return tomorrow for the actual transfusion. Alicia never ceases to amaze us all, because although we were told she would be needing a transfusion every other week during radiation, we successfully evaded another transfusion! She is not expected back at to clinic until Monday. She is due for a 2 day cycle on Monday and Tuesday, but will be doing a 5 day cycle next week. Her particular chemotherapy protocol takes into account radiation therapy, and the interaction of the drugs from the two day chemotherapy cycle. We will be in for all of next week (more ambulance rides), but this will free up July 4th week. This is when she will do her next 2 day cycle. Alicia was a bit concerned about being in the hospital for July 4th. She doesn't want to miss out on any parties! Can you blame her?

So to all those cooks out there who bring food up to the hospital, I will be letting you know what food her Royal Princess will be needing next week.

Hope everyone is well!
Rene & Alicia
(The tired ones!)

Subject: Alicia Update June 12
06/12/2002 1:03:50 PM Eastern Daylight Time

Alicia is doing well, although the radiation is making her a little tired. She is being transported via ambulance each day to LIJ, which does break up the day for her. She has been getting tutored at the hospital and she is looking forward to J.J. spending the day with her tomorrow.

It's Wednesday already, and she gets home on Saturday!
Rene & Alicia

NURSES AND DOCTORS ARE YOUR FRIENDS . . .

I AM A very social person, always have been and probably always will be. When they say the fruit doesn't fall far from the tree, it is easy to understand that my children's ability to start conversations and then have lengthy ones of substance is natural. From the beginning of treatment, Alicia was very capable of speaking directly with the nurses and doctors that cared for her. Many times, it seemed as though I was just there to keep Alicia company as she explained her history, her symptoms, and even what medications she needed to the staff. Everyone quickly grew to love her and appreciate her. She was an excellent patient who always did as she was told, never whined or complained and engaged everyone, including the cleaning people, in jovial conversation. Because of her sunny disposition, her room became a regular "hangout" for staff. During their breaks, many of them would be found sitting next to Alicia's bed, playing cards, doing crafts, or doing their nails. One day, Alicia decided to play a trick on one of the nurses named Kelly who always would joke around with Alicia. Alicia cut a small lock of hair from Lauren's head and attached it onto a piece of surgical tape. She then waited for Kelly to come into her room, and Alicia placed the piece of tape over her eyebrow. When Kelly walked in Alicia said, "Kelly, look, I am going to wax my eyebrows," and pulled the tape from her face. Of course, there was hair on it, and Kelly almost fell over. She really believed for a split second that Alicia had waxed her eyebrow. Alicia, Lauren, Kelly, and I laughed so hard we almost cried. It was a perfect example of the relationship Alicia had forged with the staff.

Their love for Alicia was exemplified one day when Alicia was out for radiation. The staff decorated her room with streamers, decorations, stickers, nail polish, cookies, candies, and a large array of kid-friendly things with a big sign that read Welcome Back Alicia. Alicia was thrilled when she returned from radiation to this wonderful display. The staff not only made Alicia's day extra special with their kindness, they showed me the power of their commitment to their patients. These were the people on the front lines of her treatment and the treatment of numerous other patients. They were the example of caregivers going above and beyond the call of duty, and they were making a difference one patient at a time. They were the silver lining of cancer's black cloud.

Subject: Alicia Update June 13
06/13/2002 11:36:37 AM Eastern Standard Time

Alicia had a tough night. She woke up at 3 AM with severe leg pain in the bone under her knee. We got her Tylenol and rubbed in until she went back to sleep, but the rest of the night was restless for her (the mother as well). Her oncologist was here early this morning to check her out and thinks the pain was caused by the Aranesp (the medication that increases her red cell production), but we will be watching her carefully.

We were picked up at 10 AM for radiation and were back at North Shore by 10:50 AM. When we returned to her room, the nursing staff had set up a whole display of cookies, candies, stickers and nail polish with a big "Welcome Back Alicia" sign. The "mayor" was very pleased.

Her chemotherapy is already hung and J.J. is here to play with her for the day. Tonight Nanny stays over so the mother can go home. (I think I need to get home for awhile)

Hope everyone is well
Rene & Alicia

Subject: Alicia Update June 17
06/17/2002 12:07:21 PM

Alicia came home fairly early on Saturday from the hospital. After a quick stop at Toys 'R Us and the addition of a Barbie laptop computer, Alicia was ready to play and get back to her life. (I hate to admit it, but her social life is much more exciting than mine.)

This morning she had radiation and is spending the day at my folk's house. Lauren had a final this morning and is spending the day with her friend. J.J. is in school. Gee, this gives me a "free" day, what shall I do? (Maybe I need to reintroduce my credit cards to the stores, LOL). With only three more day s of radiation to go, at least there is some light at the end of one tunnel!

Hope all is well
Rene & Alicia

Subject: Alicia Update June 19
06/19/2002 4:13:21 PM Eastern Standard Time

Alicia went to clinic today and for radiation. Thank goodness tomorrow is the last day of radiation. Everyday gets more tiring. Alicia wanted Lauren to see how radiation was done, since she had not gone with us yet, so both she and J.J. went with us today.

Her numbers are still okay, and we are looking forward to a good weekend. We might even "camp" in the yard and sleep in the tent. (Even though I have done that before, I'm not sure I'll be doing that now! LOL)

I am trying to attach some photos from radiation. If you can get them great, if you can't, well you know the story.

Be well
Rene & Alicia

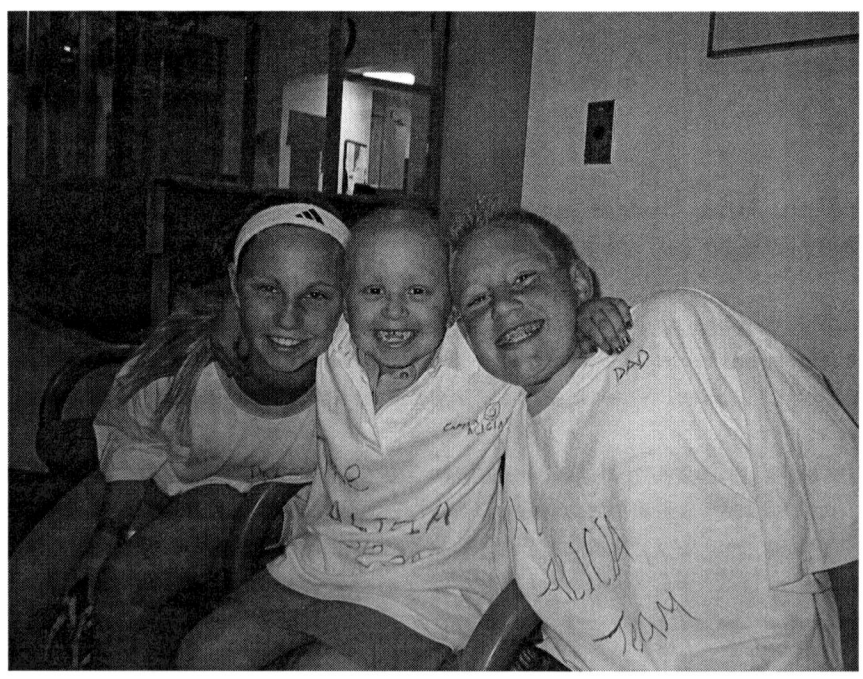

Subject: Alicia Update June 23
06/23/2002 10:12:52 PM Eastern Standard Time

Alicia finished up radiation treatment on Thursday and has been celebrating ever since. The staff at LIJ had a little sending off party for her. They were happy her treatment was completed, but sad not to see her everyday. There is something refreshing about a 6 year old skipping rope through the hallways of a hospital. To insure that she will return to visit, they gave us a new parking pass good until October

Alicia is feeling okay, although she has more fatigue and nausea. Hopefully, now that radiation is done, these symptoms will subside over time.

We are due back at clinic this week, and Alicia is going to try to go to school the last 2 days.

Hope everyone enjoyed the weekend!
Rene & Alicia

Subject: Alicia Update June 27
06/27/2002 10:07:09 AM Eastern Standard Time

We went to clinic today expecting to be in and out with just a numbers check. Unfortunately, Alicia has developed a cough that is causing her to wheeze. Possibly asthma, but they're not sure. She had to go for a chest x-ray to check her lungs. (This child glows in the dark with all the radiation and x-rays she's had.) Fortunately, her lungs are clear, but they needed to put her on an inhaler and an additional antibiotic. I am running out of fingers and toes to count all the meds she is on. LOL.

Of course this caused more time in the hospital than the mother wished to spend, especially since we had plans to go to the beach with some friends. We did get out at a reasonable time though, and did get to go to the beach. We are being admitted Monday morning for an overnight chemotherapy cycle. We have to be at oncology clinic at 8AM for port access and she has an echocardiogram at 8:30 AM. Needless to say we will be up VERY early. I thought summer meant sleeping late? LOL

Hope everyone is well and enjoys their weekend.
Rene & Alicia

Subject: Alicia Update July 8
07/08/2002 12:55:08 PM Eastern Standard Time

Alicia has been very busy since she got discharged last Tuesday. Bar-b-cues, a boat ride and basic fun. (It's a shame youth is wasted on the young, LOL.) Fourth of July, although very hot was a fun day. The highlight of the evening was our massive fireworks display (the ones we drove to Pennsylvania for). My personal favorites were my snakes (nobody else appreciated them).

Although she is a little more tired, with a schedule like hers what do you expect, she is a trouper. Other than an occasional upset stomach, she is doing just great!

Hope everyone is having as much fun as her!
Rene & Alicia

Subject: Alicia Update July 9
07/09/2002 1:47:12 PM Eastern Standard Time

Alicia went to clinic this morning for her weekly count check. Her red and white counts are low, as expected, and her platelet count is borderline for a transfusion. We need to go back to clinic on Friday, and if necessary, she will get a platelet transfusion then.

She is spending the day at her Nanny and Grandpa's house, and Lauren is going with her friend to the Britney Spears concert tonight. J.J. is hanging and all is well in the house of Giacalone.

Hope everyone is staying cool!
Rene & Alicia

Subject: Alicia Update July 12
07/12/2002 5:39:57 PM Eastern Daylight Time

Alicia had to return to clinic today for another numbers check and ended up with a platelet transfusion. Unfortunately, she has had enough of hospitals, blood tests and port accessing. I can't say I blame her, but we still have half of our chemotherapy to go and explaining this to a hysterical six year old is quite challenging. Once she was accessed, the transfusion itself was less than an hour. They took blood samples however, since her red count is low and she may need a red transfusion on Monday. We will see Monday morning.

Alicia stayed with her Nanny and Grandpa for the afternoon, which gave the frazzled mother a little break (and people wonder why I love cocktail hour, I earn it! LOL).

Till Monday, be well!
Rene & Alicia

Subject: Alicia Update July 15
07/15/2002 12:58:57 PM Eastern Daylight Time

Well we squeaked by without a red transfusion today! Whew! We brought in the "heavy hitters" though; J.J. and Alicia's friend. They were prepared to stay the whole day and keep her amused. The mother will go to any length to avoid a day like Friday. (One of the nurses started to cry today, when she was telling the social worker about Friday's accessing fiasco).

We need to go back Friday however, to make sure her numbers are good and that she is ready for Monday's admittance for 5 days of chemotherapy.

Alicia had a good weekend and looking forward to a good week.

Hope everyone is well!
Rene & Alicia

Subject: Alicia Update July 19
07/19/2002 1:57:09 PM Eastern Daylight Time

We returned to clinic yet again, and I am happy to report that Alicia did not need a red transfusion! She is expected to be admitted on Monday morning for a 5 day cycle of chemotherapy and more than likely will need a red transfusion then. This is acceptable once we are admitted; it's just the mother hates when medical treatment gets in the way of our social life. Since we have plans today, a transfusion would have been a major inconvenience. LOL.

Hope everyone has a wonderful weekend. My baby boy turns double digits on Sunday sniff, sniff. How could it be everyone else is getting older and I am not? I feel the same as when I was 19, just wished I looked that way! LOL

Be well
Rene & Alicia

Subject: Alicia Update July 22
07/22/2002 12:36:25 PM Eastern Daylight Time

Unfortunately, Alicia was unable to meet her numbers today and therefore was not admitted for chemotherapy. This cycle is exactly halfway through and her body is now starting to have a difficult time regenerating its bone marrow. Her neutrophils need to be 750 and hers were only 500. We will go back Thursday and if her numbers are good, she will be admitted then. This will have her in over the weekend, but we will deal with it.

This will now change the rest of her chemo schedule, but we have been fortunate that this hasn't happened sooner. For all my volunteers who were keeping Lauren and J.J. busy or cooking, I'll be in touch.

I'm a little drained and need a nap! LOL

Till Thursday
Rene & Alicia

Subject: Alicia Update July 24
07/24/2002 4:52:16 PM Eastern Daylight Time

Alicia is doing well. We will go tomorrow morning for our numbers check and either be admitted or sent home until Monday. (The mother is actually hoping to be sent home and start all over next week.)

I wanted to share this website, put together by one of our family friends. They were kind enough to feature Alicia in their family focus section. Have to admit, not much makes me cry, the website did. (The ice princess is melting LOL).

Enjoy!
Rene & Alicia

Subject: Alicia Update July 25
07/25/2002 1:05:27 PM Eastern Daylight Time

Alicia did not make her numbers again and was not admitted. This is good, since she will be home for the weekend. We all know how much we LOVE the weekend! I will inject her with Neupogen (for her white count) for the next three days, and then we will try again Monday. She is excited to be home, as is the mother, and we will spend the afternoon boating with her friends. What could be bad?

I will be in touch, to figure out next week's schedule, with all my volunteers.

As a side note, only 5 more months till Christmas! Thought you'd all like to know that!

Have a great day!
Rene & Alicia

Subject: Alicia Update July 30
07/30/2002 10:23:24 PM Eastern Daylight Time

We are plugging along with Alicia's chemotherapy. With the summer here however, the last place a six year old wants to be is in the hospital. The mother is going to extraordinary lengths to keep the patient upbeat. Unfortunately, it's tiring the heck out of the mother! LOL

Tomorrow is Wednesday though, and Saturday is just a few days away.

This is chemo cycle number 9, only 8 more to go!!!!!!!!!!!!!

Hanging tough!
Rene & Alicia

Subject: Alicia Update July 31
07/31/2002 5:02:31 PM Eastern Daylight Time

Alicia is having a good day. Her little friend has been here all day and has been playing with Alicia. We finally got our window in room 722 (our phone number is the same) and tonight we are watching "Crossroads" the Britney Spears movie. What could be bad?

It's Wednesday already and the weekend is just around the corner!!!!

Be well
Rene & Alicia

STATISTICS AND OTHER THINGS
THAT JUST DON'T MAKE SENSE

WHEN YOUR CHILD is diagnosed with cancer, the first question that pops into your mind is, will my child die? This is a basic and logical question that cannot be answered in a simple way. There are numerous factors that can contribute to one's outcome. The type of cancer, since some forms are more aggressive than others; where it is located and whether or not it is operable; whether the disease has metastasized, which means if it has *spread*, to other parts of the body. These, plus many additional factors, are things that all must be considered when looking at the outcome of treatment. Unfortunately, as a parent, these variables make it so extremely difficult to determine that one learns the strength of faith and prayer. One of the first things I found myself wrestling with was these numbers; the percentages of those children who live and those who die. These numbers, while seemingly easy to comprehend as just numbers, carry a much more ominous meaning when it is your child and her future they refer to. Alicia's cancer was an aggressive form of bone cancer, and while the survival rate of 75 percent would be fabulous odds in Las Vegas, they are not that reassuring when speaking about your child. My mind was already wrestling with the statistic that she was the one of the forty children per year in the United States that presented with this type of cancer in the location she did. How are those for odds? If we could win the lottery with those odds, that would have been great; however, we got cancer. My resolve from initial diagnosis and throughout her treatment was *not* to focus on those statistics, not worry about numbers and just focus on her and her health. The statistics told a certain story. I was determined to tell our own story; one that we would define the outcome on our own terms.

SOME THINGS ARE BEYOND OUR CONTROL

DURING THE SUMMER of Alicia's treatment 2003, while I was hosting bar-b-cues, driving to Pennsylvania to get Alicia sparklers for July 4 and bringing her to Hersheypark so she could have fun at an amusement park, there were those children who were not that lucky to be enjoying life like Alicia was. Alicia's little roommate, who was with us when she first got diagnosed, was one of those children. She had a form of leukemia that gave her good odds of beating her cancer. A 98 percent survival rate seemed like a gift at the time of diagnosis. Unfortunately, this quickly turned as she did not respond to her treatment, and the cancer started ravaging her young body. She was part of that 2 percent statistic that does not survive her cancer. She was a reminder that the odds can be cruel. Even after a bone marrow transplant that required an entirely new set of issues, concerns, and risks, the initial jubilation as to her prospects quickly were extinguished when the cancer returned and with more of a vengeance than before. She was going to die, and while the doctors were going to do everything in their power to prolong her life, it would be for a few weeks, maybe a few months. Not much more beyond that since her body was losing its ability to fight off her cancer as it grew weak and frail.

Alicia was in for chemotherapy when her friend and former roommate was admitted to the hospital. She was put in the room alongside Alicia, as she needed to be isolated due to her compromised immune system, and this family now had to prepare for her to die. I remember this evening very vividly as I kept asking the psychologist and social worker from the pediatric oncology unit how this could be happening since the survival statistics were so much in her favor. They reminded me that while 98 percent of patients do survive, there is the 2 percent who don't. They too make up the population of that cancer. As unfair as it was, that is how the statistic worked. I decided that evening I didn't want to *hear* about any statistics. I didn't want to hear anything about what could have or should have happened. I now had to wrestle with my thoughts that reminded me Alicia could be dealt the same cruel blow that this other family was now faced with.

Subject: I'm asking for your prayers!
07/31/2002 7:29:03 PM Eastern Daylight Time

As I sit and write my updates on Alicia, I always try to put things in a positive light. What's the point in being negative when it's so much more rewarding being upbeat. I don't want to minimize our predicament. I truly understand the seriousness of cancer, but I do feel blessed. Alicia has a good prognosis and we do our best to live life to the fullest. Everyone has been fantastic with their support and their prayers and for that I'm eternally grateful!

Having said all that, I am now asking for your prayers for a friend of Alicia's. Sarah (12 years old) was Alicia's roommate a few times. She was diagnosed with leukemia in February and had a bone marrow transplant in May. She was doing great. Unfortunately, this past week, she has taken a turn for the worst. She is being admitted this evening with a fever and will start another round of chemo on Monday. They have only given her a couple of months to live. Her mother called me with the bad news today. Her parents are making funeral arrangements for her on Saturday and they need all our prayers. I am usually never at a loss for words, but I am speechless. I don't know how to console a parent who's preparing for their child's death. So the next time your kids piss you off and you feel like yelling at them, hug them instead and please keep Sarah and her family in your prayers!

Rene

Subject: Alicia Update August 4
08/04/2002 11:07:07 PM Eastern Daylight Time

Alicia was discharged on Saturday, which marked the halfway point of her chemotherapy. Only 8 more to go! Although, it was an emotionally draining week, we tried to make the best of it as usual. The mother refuses to let anything stand in the way of a positive attitude, even if it pushes me over the edge! LOL

Both Saturday and Sunday night we had our driveway movies. We show films against our garage door and people from the neighborhood sit outside to watch. The kids had sleepovers and swam most of the weekend.

All is well on Honeysuckle Court!
Rene & Alicia

RENE A. FESLER

Subject: Alicia Update August 7
08/07/2002 11:09:58 AM Eastern Daylight Time

Alicia went to clinic this morning and her counts are low as expected. Unfortunately, she has developed fever sores all over her lips, which is really not a very good thing when your immune system is compromised. We have a prescription for Acyclovir and she needs to be watched carefully. Any fever or spreading of the sores will land us back admitted to the hospital for intravenous antibiotics. They are making me call every day until our expected return on Monday.

Keep your fingers crossed, another hospital stay does not fit into the schedule!

Be well
Rene & Alicia

Subject: Alicia Update August 9
08/09/2002 11:27:56 AM Eastern Daylight Time

Alicia is doing fine. We avoided another clinic visit because her fever sores are getting better. The acyclovir helped prevent them from spreading. Her spirits are good and she is looking forward to another good weekend.

We are going to the beach this afternoon with our friends, boating is in the plan, and there is another birthday party on Sunday.

We return to clinic on Monday. What could be bad?

Enjoy your weekend.
Rene & Alicia

Subject: Alicia Update August 12
08/12/2002 1:24:19 PM Eastern Daylight Time

Alicia did well at clinic today and is not expected back until next Monday when she will be admitted for a two day chemo cycle. She will have a bone scan and CAT scan done while admitted. I will Schedule an open MRI this week with her Uncle John and hopefully all tests will show NOTHING!

The weekend was fabulous filled with fun, friends and movies. It just goes too quickly.

Hoping everyone is well
Rene & Alicia

Subject: Alicia Update August 14
08/14/2002 10:09:32 PM Eastern Daylight Time

Alicia went for her MRI today at her Uncle John's office. The highlight of the visit was playing with John's daughter Candice. The two girls were trying to catch a goldfish out of a fish tank (and you thought a Dr's office was boring LOL).

The word is the MRI looks good. John called me this evening with the results and has sent her films to a neuroradiologist at Stony Brook University Hospital. His philosophy, you never have too many eyes looking at films. Now we just need to wait and see on her bone scan and CAT scan next week.

Alicia has spent the past 2 nights at her Nanny and Grandpa's house. Alicia said she feels like she is on a trip and will be home at the end of her trip. I think she just needs a little quiet time. We are looking forward to a quiet few days, since we don't return to the hospital until Monday when she will be admitted.

Hope everyone is doing well.

Enjoy your weekend, I know we will!
Rene & Alicia

Subject: Alicia Update August 19
08/19/2002 3:37:42 PM Eastern Daylight Time

Alicia is admitted to room 721 with a window (of course on a 2 day stay a window isn't a problem LOL). We almost did not get admitted due to low numbers. When it was suggested that we could possibly return on Thursday, the mother vehemently objected and said it wouldn't happen. We are going to Hershey Park on Friday with friends for the weekend, and NOTHING is getting in the way of fun! Even chemo needs to be flexible when it comes to a mini-vacation. She is presently resting in her room awaiting her chemotherapy.

I will be attending a North Shore fundraising event this evening, and while I was supposed to be returning home afterwards, I negotiated myself into a night of non-sleep at Club North Shore! Something I have learned, never make a deal you cannot honor and what's one more night, considering Alicia let them access her without even a tear. (She did give lots of commentary; gee I wonder where she gets that from?)

Tomorrow she is due for a CAT scan and bone scan, and then hopefully we are on our way home!!

Hope everyone is well.
Rene & Alicia

Subject: Alicia Update August 20
08/20/2002 2:54:49 PM Eastern Daylight Time

Last night upon returning from the fundraiser, I was met in the parking lot by our dear friends Maureen and her daughter Cassie. They were on their way to visit and play with Alicia, which is always a pleasant distraction.

Alicia was discharged this afternoon, but without her bone scan and CAT scan. The scheduling department had planned on the CAT scan tonight and the bone scan tomorrow night. (The mother had no intention of spending one additional second in the hospital, especially after a night of NO sleep.) Her oncologist said it was not written in stone, when these tests could be done and with a negative MRI we could do it during her next five day cycle.

Of course Alicia was fabulous with no complaints. She is already out playing and enjoying being home. They say there is no place like home and boy can we attest to that!

We are going away for the weekend and due back at clinic on Tuesday.

Enjoy your weekend
Rene & Alicia

Subject: (no subject)
08/26/2002 8:11:28 PM Eastern Daylight Time

Although I don't know who wrote this, I believe this e-mail that someone sent me has a great message.

Some years ago, on a hot summer day in South Florida, a little boy decided to go for a swim in the old swimming hole behind his house. In a hurry to dive in the cool water, he ran out the back door, leaving behind shoes, socks, and shirt as he went.

He flew into the water, not realizing that as he swam toward the middle of the lake, an alligator was swimming toward the shore.

His mother in the house was looking out the window saw the two as they got closer and closer together. In utter fear, she ran toward the water, yelling to her son as loudly as she could. Hearing her voice, the little boy became alarmed and mad a U-turn to swim to his mother. It was too late. Just as he reached her, the alligator reached him.

From the dock, the mother grabbed her little boy by the arms just as the alligator snatched his legs. That began an incredible tug of war between the two.

The alligator was much stronger than the mother, but the mother was much too passionate to let go. A farmer happened to be driving by, heard her screams and raced from his truck, took aim and shot the alligator.

Remarkably, after weeks and weeks in the hospital, the little boy survived. His legs were extremely scarred by the vicious attack of the animal, and on his arms were deep scratches where his mother's fingernails dug into his flesh in her effort to hang onto the son she loved.

The newspaper reporter, who interviewed the boy after the trauma, asked if she would show him his scars. The boy lifted his pant legs, and then with obvious pride he said to the reporter, "But look at my arms. I have great scars on my arms too. I have them because my mom wouldn't let go."

You and I can identify with that little boy. We have scars too; not from an alligator, or anything quite so dramatic, but the scars from a painful past. Some of those scars are unsightly and have caused us deep regret, but some wounds my friend, are because God refused to let go. IN the midst of your struggle, He's been holding onto you.

The Scripture teaches us that God loves you. You are a child of God. He wants to protect you and provide for you in every way, but sometimes we foolishly wade into dangerous situations. The swimming hole of life is filled with peril-and we forget that the enemy is waiting to attack. That's when the tug-of-war begins-and if you have the scars of His love on your arms, be very grateful. He did not want and will not let you go.

Subject: Alicia Update August 27
08/27/2002 1:38:11 PM Eastern Daylight Time

Alicia had a fabulous weekend at Hershey Park with her friends. She went on rides, swam and generally had a good time. The mother's philosophy, social life and mental outlook are half the battle. The busier we keep her, the less time she has to feel sorry for herself.

We went to clinic today and squeaked our way out of a red transfusion. (When the numbers are so close, the mother opts on the side of wait and see.) Her oncologist upped her dosage of Aranesp (for red count) and wants her injected today instead of tomorrow. I will be watching her for the next few days to see if she is getting lethargic. If she is, we will return to clinic this week for a transfusion. If not, we will return next Tuesday.

We are spending our last week of the summer preparing for the start of school. (The mother is always so sad to see school start. I miss having a house full of crazy kids!) Alicia is planning on attending school the first few days and meeting all her new classmates.

Her next chemo cycle is scheduled for September 16. We are putting it off by a week since we will be attending a 3 day trip out at Montauk (September 11-13) with the pediatric oncology group from North Shore.

Hope everyone is well enjoying the last of summer!
Rene & Alicia

Subject: (no subject)
09/03/2002 9:50:31 AM Eastern Daylight Time

Someone sent me this and while I don't know who wrote it, I like it.

I am thankful for . . .

The child who is not cleaning his room, but is watching TV because that means he is at home and not on the streets.

For the taxes I pay, because it means that I am employed.

For the mess to clean after a party, because it means that I have been surrounded by friends.

For the clothes that fit a little too snug, because it means I have enough to eat.

For the shadow that watches me work, because it means I am in the sunshine.

For a lawn that needs mowing, windows that need cleaning, and gutters that need fixing, because it means I have a home.

For all the complaints I hear about the government, because it means I have freedom of speech.

For the parking spot I find at the far end of the parking lot, because it means I am capable of walking and that I have been blessed with transportation.

For the huge heating bill, because it means I am warm

For the lady behind me in church that sings off key, because it means that I can hear.

For the pile of laundry and ironing, because it means I have clothes to wear.

For weariness and aching muscles at the end of the day, because it means I have been capable of working hard.

For the alarm that goes off in the early morning hours, because it means that I am alive.

And finally . . .

For too much email, because it means I have friends who are thinking of me!

RENE A. FESLER

Subject: Alicia Update September 3
09/03/2002 4:55:30 PM Eastern Daylight Time

Alicia returned to clinic today for a numbers check and once again squeaked by a transfusion. 8 is the minimum number for her red count and she was at 8. (The mother gave her iron and an Aranesp shot this morning!) We will do anything to avoid a transfusion, especially now with the talk of West Nile Virus finding it's way into the blood supply; yet another thing for the mother to obsess over.

The highlight of the weekend was Alicia mastering riding her bicycle without training wheels. (This could explain why her legs are all bruised.) She had a great weekend and is excited about the start of school tomorrow. (The mother is sad and doesn't know what she will do by herself all day.) Alicia will be attending school whenever she is up to it. The reality though, once infectious diseases start making the rounds in school, she is done.

Lauren and J.J. went for school haircuts and Alicia was so upset she wasn't getting one. Not a problem though, we just had her fuzz trimmed. She was so excited to be like the other kids, hopefully someone will notice.

We are trying to make things as "normal" as possible. I just never realized how much effort is involved trying to be like everyone else when you're dealing with cancer. LOL.

Here's to a good school year!
Rene & Alicia

Subject: Alicia Update September 6
09/06/2002 5:05:05 PM Eastern Daylight Time

Alicia attended the first three days of school and was very happy. She lasted the entire day and got her homework done quickly. She will go to clinic Monday morning and then be dropped off at school and Tuesday the oncology staff will be doing a presentation to her class.

Next Wednesday through Friday we will be going out to Montauk with other oncology families for a mini-vacation. The following Monday (9/16) Alicia is scheduled for her 5 days of chemo, but the mother is negotiating these days to allow Alicia to go to Adventure land with her school. (I have learned almost everything is negotiable! LOL)

Be well and have a great weekend!
Rene & Alicia

Subject: Alicia Update September 10
09/10/2002 5:22:38 PM Eastern Daylight Time

Alicia went to clinic on Monday without incident. She returned to school for the afternoon (she tried to negotiate her way back home) and Tuesday some of the oncology staff from North Shore did a presentation to Alicia's class.

Tonight we will be leaving for Montauk, after J.J.'s ice hockey practice. We are all looking forward to a few days away from all the insanity that has been our life this past year. We are expected to return on Friday, the mother hoping she might hit the outlets for some shopping on the way back. LOL.

Alicia will be admitted Sunday morning for the start of 5 days of chemotherapy. This will allow her to be discharged on Friday and the opportunity to participate in the Adventure land outing with her school Friday night.

We hope life is treating you all well. Tomorrow (September 11) while you are going about your day, think and pray for all the victims of that horrific day a year ago. Life does change in an instant!

Lots of Love
Rene & Alicia

Subject: Alicia Update September 14
09/14/2002 10:12:08 PM Eastern Daylight Time

We went to Montauk on Tuesday evening and returned Friday night. It was fabulous trip with something to do for everyone! (Shopping was a personal favorite of the mother). I think Lauren and J.J. had the most fun of all. Alicia enjoyed all the activities, but it was an exhausting schedule.

RENE A. FESLER

Alicia spent today riding her bicycle (two wheels) and playing with her friends. She will be admitted tomorrow morning for her 5 day chemo cycle. We need to be discharged Friday morning for her to be able to participate in Friday night's festivities at Adventure land (for my Florida friends, it's a smaller amusement park right near our house.)

I have to admit, it's getting tougher each time to pack up and know we are stuck in the hospital for a week. Cancer world is really a terrible place to live in. As we say daily, CANCER SUCKS! On the bright side, however, this is cycle number 11 of 17. We can see an end in sight.

I will be emailing photos from our Montauk trip. I didn't have a chance to download the photos since we were only home one day and I needed to take care of domestic stuff (I occasionally pretend that I am Martha Stewart). I will be emailing our room and telephone number at the hospital tomorrow.

Hope everyone is hanging tough!
Rene & Alicia

Subject: Alicia Update September 15
09/15/2002 1:03:22 PM Eastern Daylight Time

Alicia was admitted to room 719 window this morning. She started the morning off rolling around the floor complaining that she did not want to be admitted anymore and wanted to stay home. (I felt the same way, but Lauren insisted I get up off the floor LOL). I did the only thing a mother could do. I bribed her. It's amazing what some Polly Pockets can do!

Her accessing went as smooth as silk and because it was Sunday morning, the entire admission and access took about 45 minutes total! The mother is now contemplating Sunday morning admissions for the remainder of our chemo cycles.

Her blood has been drawn and we are awaiting the results of her urine tests. Hopefully, we will be ago shortly for her chemo. She is excited that Lauren and J.J. are coming to the hospital to spend the afternoon with her; she has even agreed to watch the Jet game, but more importantly the arrival of POLLY!

Hope everyone is well
Rene & Alicia

Subject: Alicia Update September 16
09/16/2002 3:14:32 PM Eastern Daylight Time

Alicia was feeling a little under the weather last night as her stomach was bothering her. Unfortunately, she was retaining too much fluid and needed Lasix to flush out her system. Obviously, this caused her to be up a lot, which meant the mother did not get much rest.

Her tutor showed up today (finally) and she got to do some school work. Lauren and J.J. are visiting this afternoon and are trying to catch up on homework they missed last week. I will be staying again this evening, oh how I miss my bed! LOL

Be well
Rene & Alicia

Subject: Alicia Update September 18
09/18/2002 9:23:10 AM Eastern Daylight Time

It's Wednesday already and Friday is just around the corner. Adventure land get ready, because here we come!

Alicia is doing well. We are monitoring her blood pressure more closely this time, as it seems to be running low and her doctors aren't sure why. Her tutor is showing up everyday (wonders never cease to exist). Unfortunately, Alicia got a roommate last night, and apparently they are handling things a little differently than us. (I think Alicia learned some new vocabulary last night!)

The mother enjoyed a good night's sleep in her own bed and actually Lauren and J.J. were never so happy to see me. (Again, wonders never cease to exist! LOL)

With the weather being so beautiful, Alicia will be taking a 'field trip' outside and around the hospital today. Gift shop here we come!

Attached to this email are some photos from our Montauk trip.

Hope you can see them. If not, I don't have a clue why.

Enjoy the day, and more importantly, enjoy your life. Life is truly wonderful, isn't it!

Be well
Rene & Alicia

(Can you tell today is a good karma day? LOL)

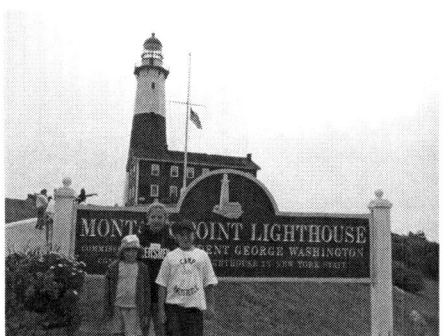
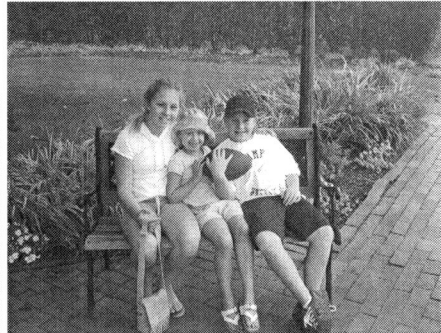

Subject: Alicia Update September 20
09/20/2002 2:36:11 PM Eastern Daylight Time

Alicia is home and ready for Adventure land this evening! She has ridden her bicycle already and is frying some snapper (freshly caught) with her Grandpa.

We got the results of her CAT scan and bone scan and I am very happy to report they were both negative!!! She had an echocardiogram this morning which also came back negative. The fluctuations in her blood pressure are an enigma to the doctors. They will be closely monitoring her throughout the rest of her chemo cycles to see if she is developing sensitivity to the medication.

No complaints here!

Hope everyone enjoys the weekend. We will be doing soccer and ice hockey with the kids and hopefully a little hot tubbing for the adults.

Be well
Rene & Alicia

Subject: Alicia Update September 23
09/23/2002 12:51:06 PM Eastern Daylight Time

Alicia had a great time at Adventure land on Friday. She went on lots of rides and was excited to see all of her friends. After a week in the hospital looking at a bunch of adults, kids were a welcomed sight.

Saturday she started soccer with her first practice, and Sunday was her first game. (They won 5-0) She played defense and offense, and wants to give being goalie a try (I need to check with the oncologist about that). J.J. played ice hockey and Lauren played soccer. I ran around like a taxicab driver! I think I need the week to rest.

Her 1st grade teacher Mrs. Caulfield will start home schooling this afternoon and my cousin Joe is coming this afternoon to perform some reflexology on the mother. I am trying desperately to maintain a positive aura!

Hope everyone's weekend was great.
Rene & Alicia

Subject: Alicia Update September 26
09/26/2002 7:54:11 AM Eastern Daylight Time

Alicia is doing well, and got out of clinic without a hitch! She spent the afternoon riding her bicycle and patiently awaiting the arrival of her tutor, Mrs. Caulfield and her 2 month old son Aidan. (He is adorable!) Our friend and Lauren's former 6th grade teacher Susan Wright stopped by to see us, and generally was a good day.

Attached to this email are forms for a North Shore pediatric cancer fundraiser. On Sunday October 27 between 1:00-4:30 there will be a bowling fundraiser. If you want to go, great; if you can't make it, not a problem. There is an additional form for sponsorship. Any money you collect will be greatly appreciated and is needed for the Children's Cancer Center. If you can't, don't worry I'll catch up to you eventually! LOL.

If you can't open the attachment, email me. They say "if at first you don't succeed, try, try again" and I will resend them. If you have any questions, call me.

Be well
Rene & Alicia

Subject: Alicia Update September 30
09/30/2002 1:27:07 PM Eastern Daylight Time

Alicia went to clinic this morning and did just fine. Her numbers are strong and we anticipate being admitted next Monday for a 2 day cycle. Hopefully, her numbers will be able to maintain themselves and we will continue on our 2 week cycle again. When you live in Cancer World however, things change constantly. (Actually, I think that's called LIFE!)

Alicia had a great weekend, as usual. She took class pictures on Friday, had a sleepover Friday night, and had soccer games both Saturday and Sunday. (of course the Honey Bees won!)

Unfortunately, going into school for visits has been cut short. It seems chicken pox has hit the elementary school and we will not take any chances. Mrs. Caulfield, her tutor, comes everyday and she has friends on the block to play with.

Some upcoming events for Alicia include her birthday, trick or treating, bowling, and an Islander game. What could be bad?

Someone posed the question, is Alicia able to be around people who get the flu shot? The answer is yes. Although she is unable to get the shot herself, other people getting it should have no impact on her.

Hope everyone is well.
Rene & Alicia

PS. Antonella-FYI we are coming into clinic next Monday for admittance. (Don't complain I didn't email you! LOL)

Subject: Alicia Update October 3
10/03/2002 12:15:39 PM Eastern Daylight Time

Alicia is doing okay, although she has picked up a case of the sniffles. The mother does not anticipate this to be a problem with Monday's chemo admittance. (I am sterilizing anyone who comes near her! LOL) She is doing well with her home tutoring and earned herself a "dinner with the teacher" the other night, for completing all her work in a timely manner (fast food as an incentive is a good thing.)

The big news in the Giacalone household is the birth of . . . baby guppies. (Shame on anyone who thought if would be anything but fish). We are quite successful in fish procreation, as this is our 3rd or 4th gaggle.)

Life is wonderful!

Enjoy
Rene & Alicia

Subject: Alicia Update October 7
10/07/2002 3:03:06 PM Eastern Daylight Time

Alicia was admitted to room 721 window. We just got up to her room now after spending 41/2 hours in clinic. (I think the nurses couldn't wait for us to leave! I know we couldn't). We were having a little problem with her urine today. Her first sample had traces of blood which needed to be investigated. Chemotherapy has just been hung, and I'm planning to bring Lauren and J.J. back tonight for a visit. (Only after I track down her Josie and the Pussycat platform shoes for Halloween costume. These are the reward for another unbelievable port accessing.) I guess the mother will be doing a lot of driving today!

Be well
Rene & Alicia

Subject: Alicia Update October 15
10/15/2002 9:16:48 PM Eastern Daylight time

Alicia has been home a week, a very good one I might add, and returned to clinic today for a numbers check. She did fabulously (we wouldn't settle for anything less) and is out visiting in the neighborhood. With her numbers being so good today, technically she is scheduled to return to the hospital on October 28 for a 5 day cycle. Of course there is a slight hitch. October 30 is her birthday and we all know what's on October 31st. The mother has officially informed the oncologist that chemo that week just won't fit into our social schedule. (Nobody ever said dealing with me was easy!) So we will be entering the hospital again on November 4 for our next cycle.

Since we all know how meek and shy the mother can be, I will now address an issue I've already introduced in a prior email. The Children's Cancer Center is holding a

Fun Bowl fundraiser on October 27th from 1:00-4:30 PM. The cost is $25 for adults and $10 for kids under 12. This includes games, shoes, lunch and soda. (There is also a Halloween costume judged contest for all who dare to dress up!)

Some of you have already notified me you will be attending. For those of you who can't come, I am hoping you will at least be a sponsor and send me a check. Any donations made will be very much appreciated and you do realize there is a tax benefit!

Remember, pediatric cancer has taken on a whole new meaning for all of us. It has a name and a face and they belong to Alicia! (Hey, I'm allowed, it's for a good cause! LOL)

Thanks to everyone
Rene & Alicia

Subject: Alicia Update October 27
10/27/2002 8:38:26 PM Eastern Standard Time

Alicia has been doing well, as usual. She had a birthday sleepover Saturday night with a few of her friends and is planning on celebrating all week long. Remember, she should be admitted for chemotherapy tomorrow, but we couldn't mess up the social plans!

Sunday was the Children's Cancer Center Fun Bowl and we all had a great time. We went with a crew of friends and family and between bowling, eating and winning prizes there was something for everyone. (The mother won a gift certificate for laser hair removal, yet I don't remember playing that raffle. LOL) actually, the highlight for the mother was winning the booby prize of "Mike's Hard Lemonade" tee shirts, the beverage of choice for our adult neighbors! Okay, I really didn't win them, I just asked for them and to get me to go away they gave them to me! LOL. Everyone sang Happy Birthday to the party girl and all shared in some birthday cake. It was a great day!

I want to thank each and every one of you in helping the Fun Bowl be such a huge success. Your support is invaluable and appreciated more than you will ever know. Just be forewarned, since I know how supportive you all are, I will be asking for you help again. I am serious and I am not shy! LOL

Thanks again
Rene & Alicia

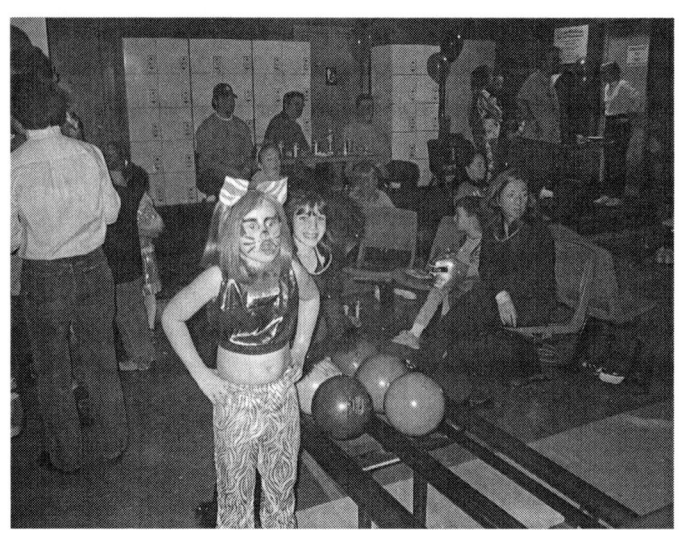

Subject: Alicia Update October 30
10/30/2002 11:22:57 AM Eastern Daylight Time

Today is . . . Alicia's birthday!!! Hard to believe she's now 7! Where did the time go? (I'm too young to have a 7 year old! LOL) So far she's having a great day, what could be bad when you are opening presents at 6:30 AM? She is feeling good and just enjoying, a valuable lesson for all to follow.

Anyone who would like to email her birthday greetings please do, she loves getting email.

Be well and take time to smell the roses!
Rene, the young mother and Alicia the 7 year old

Subject: Something to ponder
11/03/2002 9:28:08 Eastern Standard Time

Another great e-mail someone sent me. Author unknown.

Rose

The first day of school, our professor introduced himself and challenged us to get to know someone we didn't already know. I stood up to look around when a gentle hand touched my shoulder. I turned around to find a wrinkled, little old lady beaming up at me with a smile that lit up her entire being.

She said, "Hi handsome. My name is Rose. I'm eighty seven years old. Can I give you a hug?" I laughed and enthusiastically responded, "Of course you may!" And she gave me a giant squeeze. "Why are you in college at such a young, innocent age?" I asked.

She jokingly replied, "I'm here to meet a rich husband, get married, and have a couple of kids . . ." "No seriously," I asked. I was curious what may have motivated her to be taking on this challenge at her age. "I always dreamed of having a college education and now I'm getting one!" She told me.

After class we walked to the student union building and shared a chocolate milkshake. We became instant friends. Every day for the next three months we would leave class together and talk nonstop. I was always mesmerized listening to the "time machine" as she shared her wisdom and experience with me. Over the course of the year, Rose became a campus icon and she easily made friends wherever she went. She loved to dress up and she reveled in the attention bestowed upon her from the other students. She was living it up. At the end of the semester, we invited Rose to speak at our football banquet. I'll never forget what she taught us. She was introduced and stepped up to the podium. As she began to deliver her prepared speech, she dropped her three by five cards on the floor. Frustrated and a little embarrassed she leaned into the microphone and simply said, "I'm sorry. I'm so jittery. I gave up beer for lent and this whiskey is killing me! I'll never get my speech back in order so let me just tell you what I know."

As we laughed, she cleared her throat and began, and we do not stop playing because we are old' we grow old because we stop playing; there are only four secrets to staying young, being happy and achieving success."

"You have to laugh and find humor everyday. You've got to have a dream. When you lose your dreams, you die. We have so many people walking around who are dead and don't even know it! There is a huge difference between growing old and growing up. If you are nineteen years old, lie in bed for one full year, and don't do one productive thing and you will turn twenty years old. I am eighty seven years old and stay in bed for a year and never do anything I will turn eighty eight. Anybody can grow older. That doesn't take any talent or ability. The idea is to grow up always finding the opportunity in change.

Have no regrets. The elderly usually don't have regrets for what we did, but rather for things we did not do. The only people who fear death are those with regrets."

She concluded her speech by courageously singing "The Rose." She challenged each of us to study the lyrics and live them out in our daily lives.

At the years end Rose finished the college degree she had begun all those years ago.

One week after graduation, Rose died peacefully in her sleep. Over two thousand college students attending her funeral in tribute to the wonderful woman who taught by example that it's never too late to be all you can possible be.

These words have been passed along in loving memory of Rose.

Remember, growing older is mandatory. Growing up is optional. We make a living by what we get; we make a life out of what we give. God promises a safe landing, not a calm passage. If God brings you to it, he will bring you through it.

Subject: Alicia Update November 4
11/04/2002 1:16:37 PM Eastern Standard Time

Alicia is admitted to room 719 door (we will be moved to a window shortly.) She let them access her port with a minimal amount of tears and is currently awaiting the start of chemotherapy. I truly am amazed at the courage and strength continuously exhibited by this child. I just wish I was as strong as her. She is presently working on a sewing project and is looking forward to tomorrow when Lauren, J.J. and a friend of hers will come to spend the day.

Her chemotherapy is action packed, as usual, and we are seeing and end in sight to chemotherapy. This our 13th cycle with only 1 more 5 day admittance after this week and 3 2 day admittances.

Life is good!
Rene & Alicia

Subject: Alicia Update November 5
11/05/2002 1:59:23 PM Eastern Standard Time

Alicia is doing okay. She is experiencing low blood pressure at night that she had the last time we were admitted for her 5 day cycle. This cycle, she has been getting a reconfigured formula of etoposide, the drug that seems to be causing the difficulty, but we still seem to be having some trouble. Her chemo for today has yet to be hung, and she is presently playing Polly Pockets with J.J. and a friend. Lauren is enjoying doing arts and crafts and the mother is experiencing a sugar overload due to too much Halloween candy

Some of our friends, Nanny Fran and Poppy John came in for a surprise visit which is always a welcome treat. Later this evening, Nanny and Grandpa will be here and the mother will be taking the kids from Honeysuckle Court back to the block. If all goes well, I will be spending the night at home, but a drop in blood pressure could cause a late night run back to the hospital. Let's hope all goes well.

Be well
Rene & Alicia

Subject: Alicia Update November 7
11/7/2002 5:03:14 PM Eastern Standard Time

Alicia is plugging along as usual. Last night we didn't experience low blood pressure, we experienced high blood pressure. It is said that life is full of ups and downs, well so is blood pressure. LOL

After the mother had left for home this afternoon, Alicia was going on a "field trip" to the gift shop. Saturday is Lauren's birthday and you know Alicia can always use a little something herself! Tonight Nanny gets to stay at the hospital. Tomorrow Alicia will get to watch "Meet the Parents" for the 15th time and Saturday Her Royal Highness will return home and round 13 is over!

Life is good!
Rene & Alicia

LIFE IS NOT FAIR . . .

THE TONE OF Alicia's treatment, as can be witnessed through these e-mails, was one of a dedicated perseverance to conquer her cancer. Living life to the fullest and enjoying ourselves along the way lulled me into a false sense of "security." I immersed myself in her treatment, care and having an incredibly interesting life, so I was able to block out of my mind most of the time the devastation cancer can and does inflict. A vibrant and happy child could not be one who would die; or at least I tried to convince myself.

My philosophy about life is fairly simple and straightforward. While I tried to be truthful yet positive and upbeat, the devastation of cancer was always right around the corner. My life and my view of the world changed on November 9. It was on this day I learned that even with the best medical treatment, the most positive attitude, and the most loving family surrounding someone, cancer is cruel. Another victim was taken, another family was crushed, and it just wasn't fair!

Subject: Please say a prayer
11/09/2002 11:59:53 PM Eastern Standard Time

I've spent the past 10 months writing emails about Alicia's progress. Beating her cancer has been our sole mission and the road we still travel on. We have been hell bent on living life and having fun. Were we always like this or has her cancer given us a different perspective on what is truly important?

Having cancer puts you into a totally different realm of existence that I call Cancer World. The citizens of this culture are ordinary people faced with extraordinary circumstances. You do not have a choice of whether or not you want to join, you are drafted. When you enter this world, life as you once knew it has changed. A good percentage of its citizens respond well to treatment and are "cured" of their cancer. There are however, percentages that don't. Unfortunately, one of Alicia's former roommates Sarah joined the percentage of those who don't, when she passed away today. I cannot even begin to express the sadness felt in my heart, not only for the loss of a 12 year old little girl, but for a family left behind who has to deal with this tragedy. In an ironic twist of fate, we spent the day celebrating Lauren's 13th birthday and Alicia's return home from the hospital, while Sarah's family watched their daughter die. The blessing in this, if there is one, was she wasn't in any pain, a small comfort at such a horrific time.

I have had numerous discussions with cancer families as to why things happen and the meaning to such God awful heartache. Unfortunately, there is never an answer. I don't know why Alicia got cancer, and I don't know why God chose Sarah to die. What I do know though is all of you have an opportunity to learn from our heartache. Really treasure your lives and never take anything for granted. If you are blessed enough to have your health and people around you who love you, cherish them as though they were gold. Never take anyone for granted. Tell your husband/wife and children how much you love them and live life to the fullest!

Listen more, complain less and appreciate the most. Make a difference in your life and don't let our heartache be for naught!

May Sarah rest in Peace.
Rene

Subject: Life goes on
11/13/2002 12:46:18 PM Eastern Standard Time

The past few days have been difficult for our family as we have tried to come to terms with Sarah's passing. Life does go on however, and we have to keep on living. If we let cancer, death or any other obstacle paralyze us in our lives, we have given it more power than it is worthy of.

I apologize to those of you who found yourselves crying reading my last email. I much prefer being the court jester to the philosopher. For your information, I did tell Alicia about Sarah's passing. I made a pact with her when she was first diagnosed that I would never lie to her about what was going on. We needed to trust each other and I would explain everything to her regarding her treatment, and let her know what to expect every step of the way. I couldn't lie to her now. As expected, she was very sad, but felt honored that Sarah was buried with a gift Alicia had given her on one of her "field trips" to the hospital gift shop. In usual Alicia style though, she made me feel better with her words and maybe you'll think so too.

"Sarah is an angel living with God now. Most people have to live their whole lives to get there. Sarah's there now. Isn't she lucky?"

Here's to living!
Rene

Subject: Alicia Update November 18
11/18/2002 3:25:04 PM Eastern Standard Time

Alicia is doing well. Friday was filled with a clinic visit with her friends in tow. (The elementary school had off), lunch at the diner and an evening with "Harry Potter." The rest of the weekend was the standard playing with friends and having fun.

This weekend she is attending a birthday celebration for the twins across the street, so this afternoon we had to do some shopping. Shopping with Alicia is a trip! She can play all day, ride her bicycle, play dolls, school, whatever. Just wheel her into a store and the "sleepy gremlin" takes over. Needless to say, other than the twin's presents, the mother got no shopping done. We did bump into one of the pediatric nurses from the hospital at Kohl's. Alicia told her she looked different in "normal" clothes. I think Alicia was surprised that nurses have lives outside of the hospital. LOL

The big news in the Giacalone household today is . . . Lauren brought home a baby! Part of the 8th grade health program is to bring home a computerized baby. It is only for overnight, thank goodness, and only Lauren is supposed to take care of her. The attitude of the teenager is classic, what a drag as she keeps on walking around the house with the baby in the infant seat saying, "I hate this!" Alicia thinks Lauren is being more of a baby than the baby. LOL

Hope everyone is well as we are edging closer to the holiday season. Do you think it's too early to start putting up our Christmas trees? We have clinic on Friday and are expected to be admitted to the hospital on Monday morning for an overnight stay. This is cycle #14 of 17. Hooray, the end is in sight!!!! Let's just keep our fingers crossed that Alicia maintains her numbers and stays on target. Although I hate to admit it, some things are just out of the mother's control!

Be well
Rene & Alicia

Subject: Alicia Update November 22
11/22/2002 3:01:12 PM Eastern Standard Time

Alicia had clinic this morning for her numbers check and in usual Alicia style, she did great! Next we did lunch, always a personal favorite. Finally, we went to her school for a re-take of her class photo and she got to spend a little time with her class. J.J. was excited I took him home early and its FRIDAY! You know what that means? Party, party, party!!!!! Remember, nothing, not even cancer, gets in the way of the social schedule! LOL

Alicia will be admitted Monday morning for an overnight stay and will get to enjoy the holiday at home. Both Alicia and Lauren are bugging me to get the Christmas decorations up; I haven't put Halloween away yet.

Hope everyone is well!
Rene & Alicia

Subject: Alicia Update November 25
11/25/2002 4:02:23 PM Eastern Standard Time

Alicia is admitted to room 721 window. She almost wasn't admitted because her numbers were a little low, but good enough for chemotherapy.

She has been selling jewelry all day to the staff. (It's a long story) She is quite persuasive and has almost run out of inventory. (Ms. Rosemary, can I get more stuff for her tonight?) This has made the day fly by.

GTG
Rene & Alicia

Subject: Alicia Update November 26
11/26/2002 3:29:56 PM Eastern Standard Time

Alicia is home, hip, hip hooray! Number 14 is done, number 15 here we come. I have to admit this stay went quite quickly. Maybe it was the fact Alicia was "hawking" jewelry the whole time. For everyone's information, we are in the process of setting up a not for profit foundation to raise money for children with cancer and their families.

We've been so blessed this year with our network of family and friends; we just want to give a little back.

We are anxiously awaiting the arrival of snow here in New York, and Lauren, J.J. and Alicia are ready to decorate for Christmas. Hopefully the snow won't disturb the Thanksgiving plans.

J.J. has a hockey tournament in Cherry Hill, New Jersey and the girls will be shopping, oh the trouble we can get into LOL.

Wishing everyone a Happy Thanksgiving!
Rene & Alicia

Subject: Alicia Update December 3
12/3/2002 3:35:15 PM Eastern Standard Time

Alicia had clinic today, with numbers that are quite remarkable if I might add. I guess the winter makes everyone look pale and is not necessarily and indication of blood counts. Lauren needed a visit with the doctor, she's got the blah's like most everyone. We did lunch at on of my old-time favorite diners, Sea crest in Old Westbury. (Brings me back to my high school hang out days which were just a few short years ago!)

Lauren is spending the afternoon with her Nanny, which caused a bit of stress for the "wee little one" aka Alicia. So what does the mother do? Suggest a trip to a local nursery called Hicks to look at Christmas trees. Guess who is now driving around with a 10 foot Christmas tree on their roof? We will need to figure out how to get this big tree into the house. Lately, I'm not sure if our life is more sitcom or soap opera.

Thanksgiving was nice and this past weekend ushered in the "official" start of Christmas decorating on Honeysuckle Court. The competition is fierce around here! LOL Over the weekend we also attended a Bat Mitzvah for our friend, and a good time was had by all as you can see from the attached pictures.

Hope everyone is well and gearing up for a spectacular holiday season. It was 1 year ago today; December 3rd that Alicia first visited her pediatrician with her backache. What a year this has been. If anyone had told me then where we would be sitting now, I would have bet my life against it. Although I can't speak for everyone, I know this year has dramatically changed who I am. Whether it is for better or for worse depends on whose perspective you are looking at it from. I am an eternal optimist, but deep down I hurt. I crave to be surrounded with positive energy, but have negative feelings myself. I am strong and determined, yet I feel frail and vulnerable. I cry like all people do, just in the privacy of my own company. I do not have all the answers, and I don't want anyone to try to be me. Each of us is unique in our own way and need to cope and find contentment in that. (LAG you are perfect just being you!)

To all of you, thank you for being you!

Love
Rene & Alicia

Subject: Alicia Update December 9
12/9/2002 3:14:35 PM Eastern Standard Time

Alicia is doing spectacularly well. We went Christmas tree cutting on Saturday with some of our friends, even some of our Jewish friends. What can I say; they are getting indoctrinated into life as per "Giacalone." Hang around with us long enough; you just might turn into us, now there's a scary thought! LOL. My personal favorite part of the day was a stop at one of the wineries for some wine tasting and the purchase of some holiday vino, followed by lunch at Bennigans. J.J. had an ice hockey game at Chelsea Pier, (they lost) and Saturday night was tree decorating and a sleepover for Alicia. Unfortunately, with such stiff competition with the outside holiday decorations on this block, we have run into the problem of overloaded circuits. (Clark Griswold watch out!)

Sunday was another busy day with shopping on the schedule, chocolate making and Lauren attending the Jet game with our neighbor Michael. Monday has arrived quickly and Alicia and I are attempting to clean up her room . . . quite an undertaking and not for the faint of heart. We are already up to 5 black garbage bags full of "stuff." We will do clinic on Wednesday, (is that okay Antonella?)And are preparing for next week's last 5 day chemo cycle . . . hip, hip, hooray! We will look to be admitted Monday and she'll be home on Saturday. We have to get more jewelry for her to sell up at the hospital and hopefully the week will fly by.

Alicia is doing very well, I marvel at her strength and stamina. She is an incredibly strong and determined little girl who refuses to let cancer get in the way of her life.

Whenever I feel a little down, I look no further than Alicia to really appreciate how lucky we are. I believe I have spoken about the foundation we are in the process of setting up to raise funds for families faced with cancer. We want other families to be able to "live" while dealing with cancer, like we have been able to do. So with this in mind, I am putting out a call to everyone for fundraising ideas and volunteers. We already have had the jewelry sale and one of my teacher friends is holding a fundraiser in her middle school. Someone suggested compiling these emails and publishing them, a cookbook was suggested and the big one I am looking into is a golf outing. So in the middle of all the holiday hustle and bustle, I am asking all of you to take a few minutes and brainstorm. Any ideas will be appreciated, and any volunteers will be appreciated even more! LOL

Be well and stay in touch
Rene & Alicia

Subject: Alicia Update December 12
12/12/02 11:06:44 AM Eastern Standard Time

Alicia was in and out of clinic yesterday in no time flat. Not to jinx her, but she appears to be rebounding from her chemo remarkably well. She spent the afternoon doing lunch with Grandpa and returned home in time to have home tutoring with Mrs. Caulfield.

She is scheduled to be admitted Monday morning for her final 5 day chemotherapy cycle (#15 of 17) YEAH! Unfortunately, trying to get the patient excited about going into the hospital the week before Christmas will require some creativity. The mother will not be able to spend as much time in the hospital since there is a holiday to plan for. Anyone who wants to visit her next week is encouraged to do so. If you can't visit, a call would be nice. Unbeknownst to her, Nanny and Grandpa bought a little Christmas tree to set up in her room (we really need that window Joann and Antonella!) We are planning on making the week even more festive than our usual stay. (Hard to imagine, I'm sure the staff will be thrilled LOL.) We need to keep the "mayor" of the 7th floor happy and we are celebrating this last 5 day stay!

Hope everyone is well and enjoying themselves. The Monday email will have both her room and telephone numbers.

Rene & Alicia

RENE A. FESLER

Subject: Alicia Update December 16
12/16/2002 4:54:02 PM Eastern Standard Time

Alicia is currently admitted to room 719 door, we will be moved in a little bit to room 722 window. This is her last 5 day cycle, number 15 of 17 HOORAY!!!!! We only got to her room around 4 PM since the census on the 7th floor is high. This was not a problem however, since the patient was once again selling her jewelry.

She had another wonderful weekend with a sleepover, pizza party and holiday decorating. We have pushed the decorating to the limit and have even decorated our single Jewish neighbor's house while he wasn't home. The holiday decorating competition has gotten so fierce that one of our neighbors distributed a letter on the block declaring a certain blonde a "traitor" who didn't honor a decorating truce. LOL.

All is well on Honeysuckle.

The mother will be spending the night and Lauren and J.J. are coming up to spend some time.

Hope everyone is enjoying this holiday season.

Rene & Alicia

Subject: Alicia Update December 17
12/17/2002 12:35:31 PM Eastern Standard Time

Alicia is doing spectacularly well. (Would we accept anything less?) Last night Lauren and J.J. were here and the three of them spent 2 hours in the playroom making Christmas ornaments. Her room is decorated with a Christmas tree, garland and lights and candy canes. She has her room set up like a jewelry store and has sent the word around the hospital that she is "open for business."

Early this morning her uncle brought Dunkin Donuts and this afternoon she will do some school work. Hopefully, the mother will be leaving this afternoon to tend to some Christmas planning. Nanny will spend this evening which should be fairly uneventful. Last night she experienced no blood pressure problems, just some leg pain. Unfortunately, in a child with bone cancer the mother's imagination runs a little wild in the middle of the night, but by morning her pain had subsided.

Only 8 more days till Christmas, and Alicia anxiously awaits the arrival of Santa

Be well
Rene & Alicia

Subject: Alicia Update December 18
12/18/2002 5:27:32 PM Eastern Standard Time

Hope this email finds everyone well. Only one more week till Christmas! Some little ones just can't wait. Let's hope no one is disappointed with Santa's selections. Alicia is sailing through this cycle of chemotherapy. I think the fact that she knows this is her last LONG stay is helping her. Today she has had numerous visitors, a big thank you to all, and she is enjoying the 'festive' mood of all the people around her.

Unfortunately, in the never ending attempt to keep our life interesting, and to give you more to read about, J.J. is home sick today. (The mother just can't get some time alone to do the Christmas stuff.) A trip to the doctor has identified his condition as a mild case of bronchitis. So now there is a good chance that he will be starting his Christmas break NOW! Ugh! Jewelry sales have slowed a bit and there is a lot of crafting going on.

Hope everyone is well and not too stressed. Remember, take time to enjoy!

Rene & Alicia

Subject: Alicia Update December 19
12/19/2002 4:41:20 PM Eastern Standard time

Thursday is here and Alicia is doing just great! So far she has been lucky and not had a roommate. Considering all of her company and the jewelry sale this is a good thing. She is feeling fine and is looking forward to coming home on Saturday. You know there is a lot of preparation for Christmas when you are 7 years old!

J.J. went with the mother to COSTCO (OH MY GOODNESS) to shop for Christmas dinner, followed by a trip to the bank and then an afternoon with Grandpa.

Candy making and wrapping presents are on tonight's home schedule. Hope everyone is prepared, only 6 more days!!!!!

Have a good night
Rene & Alicia

Subject: Alicia Update December 20
12/20/2002 2:53:46 PM Eastern Standard Time

Well it's Friday at North Shore Hospital and ALL is well. Seems Santa Claus dropped by the 7th floor today for a visit with the kids. Lots of presents for the kids, none for the parents (guess the parents weren't that good this year LOL), but the kids were happy and that is all that matters. As I type Alicia is getting the last of this particular chemo cycle. Although I am thrilled beyond words, I can't help but feel a little melancholy knowing that ALL these incredible people who have so tirelessly kept my daughter alive pretty soon will not longer be part of our routine and our lives. We have already stared exchanging phone numbers and addresses, since it is tough to see Alicia "go." Have any of you noticed how once a friend of the Giacalone's, ALWAYS a friend of the Giacalone's? We are sort of like something stuck on the bottom of your sneaker, even if you want it be gone, it's always stuck there! LOL

Alicia is at a sing-a-long in the playroom with the music therapist and the mother is just doing a little reflecting. This leads me to my next request (always an angle from me). As we are winding down our treatment, and especially at this time of year when we try to find some deeper meaning for our lives, I am asking all of you to look deep inside of yourselves and tell me how this year has changed you if it has at all. Has Alicia's cancer made any difference in your life? What do you do now differently that you didn't do a year ago? If I decide to publish my emails, let me know if I could include your email along with mine, (for my attorney friends, that counts at consent correct? LOL) numerous people have told me that this 'diary' of the past year would be so helpful to other people facing adversity (if nothing else it should help Mike's Hard Lemonade's business LOL). I will be sending out my own email with my thoughts of the past year (I will try to make a non-hanky email, but I can't make promises LOL).

Let me go enjoy the caroling

Till tomorrow, be well
Rene & Alicia

Subject: Alicia Update December 24
12/24/2002 7:32:00 AM Eastern Standard Time

*Alicia came home Saturday and completed her LAST 5 day cycle of chemotherapy!!
HIP HIP HOORAY!!!! Last year it seemed as though we would never see the end of
the long stays, yet we have.*

*Of course her weekend was typically action packed playing with friends, baking,
candy making and the Sunday night climax of the holiday decorating contest on
Honeysuckle Court. In a shameless attempt to "win" at all costs, the mother pulled
out all stops. As one friend put it, "so I hear you obtained a nuclear weapon of
decorating?" . . . We put on a live performance of the Christmas story along with
music, a narrator on a PA system, and a fog machine for special effects. At the end
of the show, the mother served hot spiced cider, hot chocolate and cookies. So did I
win? NO . . . the little cancer patient was one of the judges and gave me honorable
mention. As she put it, I didn't want to hurt the other people's feelings . . . some
heck of a kid huh?*

*We've already had our nails done for Christmas, just finishing up with some
wrapping and completing our cooking preparing for the big day! The anticipation in
the house is growing moment by moment. Let's just hope no one will be disappointed.
J.J. asked me if it's okay to ask for the impossible. He said instead of any presents
this year, he had wished and prayed that Alicia had never gotten cancer and could
just be a regular kid again. It has become quite evident to all of us that this whole
experience has matured her years well beyond her age. Her "childhood innocence"
is gone. As I told J.J., what's done is done. Never look back with sadness or regret.
We have had a year in which we got to witness and experience the goodness of
people. Alicia is doing great, and hey . . . we just got medical approval for Alicia's
wish from Make-A-Wish. LOL we are truly blessed and hopefully we will never
lose sight of that.*

*Be on the lookout for my Christmas email with possibly a video clip (I am getting real
hi tech). We want everyone to share in the "magic" of Christmas!*

*May you enjoy your time with your families and take a moment to reflect and appreciate
how lucky we all are!!!*

Merry Christmas and God Bless

Rene & Alicia

RENE A. FESLER

Subject: A Merry Christmas Wish from Rene, Lauren, J. J. & Alicia
12/25/2002 2:23:19 PM Eastern Standard Time

Here's wishing everyone a Merry Christmas and for all our Jewish friends a good movie and some great Chinese food! LOL

I believe all three Giacalone children were more than satisfied with Santa's selections this year. We are now the proud family of a Yorkshire terrier puppy named Jingle Belle. We need to follow more stringent rules with hand washing and keeping Alicia away from "poop" duty LOL, but other than that, her oncologist gave it her blessing. Let's hope this "new baby" sleeps through the night! Other gifts included clothes, dolls and a cell phone for one particular 13 year old named Lauren.

We are currently awaiting the arrival of our company and expect to have one heck of a day. Quite a change from last Christmas, so we really need to celebrate!

Merry Christmas to all!

Rene & Alicia

Subject: Alicia Update December 27
12/27/2002 2:47:30 PM Eastern Standard Time

Hope everyone's holiday was good. We had a wonderful Christmas. The snow that fell here Christmas evening made for a long commute for some of our guests, but everyone got home safe. Our new addition "Jingle Belle" is doing just fine. The kids now realize how much work a dog is since the mother is letting them do it all.

J.J. left Thursday evening for Valley Forge, PA for weekend hockey tournament. He isn't expected back until late Sunday, so that leaves me and girls home alone. Oh no!

Alicia went to clinic today and had okay numbers. We need to return Monday to monitor how she is doing. Unfortunately, the mother has gotten laryngitis and has limited speaking ability. (The kids can enjoy some silence . . . LOL). We will manage to enjoy ourselves this weekend though, and are looking forward to New Year's Eve when we are planning a balloon drop, lighted ball drop and fireworks display! Hey, after the year we've had, we are entitled to celebrate the coming of the New Year, right?

Be Well
Rene & Alicia

Subject: RE: Alicia Update December 27
12/27/2002 4:33:26 PM Eastern Standard Time

*THE MOM HAS LARYNGITIS-WE ALL WISH HER WELL-BUT THE SILENCE
IS GOLDEN!!*

*SERIOUSLY-A HAPPY HEALTHY NEW YEAR TO ALL-AND MAY ALICIA'S
ORDEAL IN 2002 FADE FAST INTO OUR COLLECTIVE MEMORIES-AND
MAY 2003 AND BEYOND HOLD NOTHING BUT HEALTH AND HAPPINESS
TO HER AND HER FAMILY!!!*

A FAMILY FRIEND

Subject: Alicia Update December 30
12/30/2002 11:39:02 AM Eastern Standard Time

*I want to take this opportunity to wish everyone a happy and more importantly
healthy New Year! I was never so glad to see a year leave as I am this year.
Although we managed to get through it, it was not without a cost. My little baby
has been robbed of her childhood that she will never get back. My eldest daughter
was forced to confront life and death just as she was entering her teenage years.
My little man turned into a bowl of mush in front of my eyes because he was so
scared his little sister was going to die. As for me, well what can be said? I went
into this optimistic for a good outcome, but also at a cost. I am not the person I
was a year ago. Circumstances have changed, and so have I. As someone put it
to me, "Rene, you have lost your 'warm and fuzzy' feeling." For that I am sorry,
but you cannot go through what we have and remain the same. I know we have
been blessed with family and friends who have stood by us and given us their
all. I feel anger though as to why we had to go through this to begin with. I
was rather enjoying just being an average middle class family when the rug was
pulled out from under our feet. So now, I don't have the patience for people who
make mountains out of mole hills and dote on minutia. I speak my mind even
more freely (hard to imagine huh?), since I really don't care if people like what I
have to say. I don't sweat the small stuff because in the scheme of things it really
doesn't matter. I have learned that it's okay to cry, but it's also okay to laugh in
the face of adversity. Never lose your sense of humor; it may be your only saving
grace when you are overcome with grief: when you have an opportunity to have*

fun, do it that moment. Never take for granted tomorrow . . . there just might not be any. Welcome change with open arms. Change is inevitable and fighting it will only cause you heartache. Believe in positive thinking, since state of mind is half the battle.

A little girl named Alicia showed us all what a positive attitude can do!

May 2003 is a better year for everyone!!!!

Rene & Alicia

Subject: Alicia Update January 2
1/2/2003 7:50:28 PM Eastern Standard Time

Not much to report, other than the fact I have spent more time running around this neighborhood in my robe after a certain puppy than I care to admit. (The mother is losing her sense of humor!). Alicia, Lauren and J.J. are all doing well. J.J. was stressing over the return to school today, but he got over it quick enough, he had no choice.

Alicia is feeling well and is expected to be admitted Monday morning for her next to last over night stay.

Some of you have requested pix of the newest addition so here are some holiday photos.

Be well
Rene & Alicia

Subject: Alicia Update January 6
Date: 1/6/2003 4:24:44 PM Eastern Standard Time

Alicia is admitted to room 719 window. We got a late start this morning since the patient was tired and needed to be woken up, then the dog got out of the yard while the mother chased her all around the neighborhood. Thank goodness my neighbor joined the posse to help catch her; otherwise I still might be chasing her!

We spent most of our day down in clinic with the lovely oncology nursing staff. (How's that girls?) Alicia did some crafts watched Cinderella and basically bossed us all around. This evening nanny will be staying since I need to tend to the puppy, and Alicia will be baking cookies in the playroom.

We are planning an early "break out" tomorrow, since we have things to do.

Hope everyone is doing well.
Rene & Alicia

Subject: Alicia Update January 7
Date: 1/7/2003 4:10:19 PM Eastern Standard Time

Cycle 16 is complete!!!!
Hard to imagine a year ago we were just starting this nightmare and here we are almost finished. What a ride this has been and Alicia as usual, is doing it with style. All the staff made a point to visit Alicia since she always makes everyone feel so good. Our room therefore was a constant parade of visitors. The roommate Alicia had was also a little girl who appeared to be on the start of her journey, and the looks of her family were curious because how could there be such joy and happiness on the pediatric floor with cancer patients? Very easy . . . just believe anything is possible! If you tell a child they can't handle something they won't. If you tell them to shoot for the stars and you know they are capable of great things, they will rise to the occasion.

Remember, we are only limited by our own fears . . . let's not import them upon our children. As we all witnessed, great things CAN be expected of little people if we just believe in them!

May we all believe in the strengths of our children!

Rene & Alicia

Subject: Alicia Update January 8
1/8/2003 2:41:37 PM Eastern Standard Time

Hope this email finds everyone well. Our little cancer patient is feeling the effects of chemo all day today. However, not one complaint from her, just a lot of resting. WE have rigged up a piece of fence to keep Jingle Belle in the yard, thank goodness

I think I've done enough running around this neighborhood (think I've frightened a few people LOL).

Want to put out a plea to all of you. If any of you have a connection at a county club that hosts charity golf outings here on Long Island, could you please get me a name and telephone number of someone to speak to at the club. The Foundation is looking to host our first annual golf outing as a fundraiser, and it always is nice to have an introduction.

Thanks for any info

Have a great day!
Rene & Alicia

Subject: Aging
1/9/2003 8:14:54 PM Eastern Standard Time

Another great e-mail from an unknown author.
Do you realize that the only time in our lives when we like to get old is when we're kids? If you're less than 10 years old, you're so excited about aging that you think in fractions. "How old are you? I'm four and a half!" You're never thirty-six and half. You're four and a half, going on five!

That's the key. You get into your teens, now they can't hold you back. You jump to the next number, or even a few ahead. "How old are you? I'm going to be 16!" You could be 13, but hey, you're going to be 16!

And then the greatest day of your life . . . you become 21. Even the words sound like a ceremony . . . YOU BECOME 21 YESSS!

But then you turn 30. Ooooh, what happened here? Makes you sound like bad milk. HE TURNED: we had to throw him out. There's no fun now, you're just a sour-dumpling. What's wrong? What's changed?

You BECOME 21, your TURN 30, then you're PUSHING 40. WHOA! Put on the brakes, it's all slipping away. Before you know it, you REACH 50 . . . and your dreams are gone.

But wait!!! You MAKE it to 60. You didn't think you would! So you BECOME 21, TURN 30, PUSH 40, REACH 50, and MAKE it to 60.

You've built up so much speed that you HIT 70! After that it's a day by day thing: you HIT Wednesday!

You get into your 80's and every day is a complete cycle; you HIT lunch; you TURN 4:30; you REACH your bedtime. And it just doesn't end there. Into your 90's you start going backwards; "I was just 92."

Then a strange thing happens. If you make it over 100, you become a little kid again. "I'm 100 and a half!"

May you all make it to a healthy 100 and a half!

HOW TO STAY YOUNG

1. Throw out all nonessential numbers. This includes age, weight, and height. Let the doctor worry about them. That is why you pay him/her.
2. Keep only cheerful friends. The grouches pull you down.
3. Keep learning. Learn more about the computer, crafts, gardening, whatever. Never let the brain idle. "An idle mind is the devil's workshop" and the devil's name is Alzheimer's.
4. Enjoy the simple things.
5. Laugh often, long and loud. Laugh until you gasp for breath.
6. The tears happen. Endure, grieve and move on. The only person who is with us our entire life is ourselves. Be ALIVE while you are alive.
7. Surround yourself with what you love, whether it's family, pets, keepsakes, music, plants, and hobbies, whatever. Your home is your refuge.
8. Cherish your health: if it is good, preserve it. If it is unstable, improve it. If it is beyond what you can improve, get help.
9. Don't take guilt trips. Take a trip to the mall, to the next county, to a foreign country, but NOT to where the guilt is.
10. Tell the people you love that you love them, at every opportunity.

AND ALWAYS REMEMBER:

Life is not measured by the number of breaths we take, but by the moments that take our breath away.

If you don't send this to at least 8 people—who cares?

Subject: Alicia Update January 13
1/13/2003 11:05:46 AM Eastern Standard Time

Alicia had a good weekend . . . unfortunately; the other Giacalone children did not. The stomach virus that has been going around has visited Lauren and today J.J. Although we have been lucky up to his point with minimizing sickness, it was necessary to send them to Nanny and Grandpa's house to recuperate. (Let's hope my parent's doing get sick.) Needless to say I feel so guilty (yes even the blonde has moments of guilt) not being able to take care of Lauren and J.J. With me being the only caregiver for Alicia, dispensing her medications and doing her injections, it was only logical that I also could not be exposed to them.

Jingle Belle is doing well . . . she got out of the backyard on Saturday which caused hysteria in the house. We almost thought she was gone for good, luckily J.J. found her in our neighbors yard. Seems a little girl who resides in this house, along with her friends, moved the makeshift gate we had and didn't place it back properly. So when we thought Jingle was "secure" in the yard, she was wandering the streets of Country Pointe. We had a good ending though, and Alicia now knows not to move the gate.

For all your Jet fans . . . better luck next year!

Hope everyone is well!
Rene & Alicia

Subject: Alicia Update January 14
1/14/2003 10:31:05 AM Eastern Standard Time

In our never ending attempt to keep everyone amused . . . another family member has fallen ill to the terrible stomach virus (I'm just glad it's not me! LOL). The husband arrived home early from work and retired to bed for the evening. Can you believe he wanted me to tend to him??? I did throw him his cell phone and a few water bottles from the door! Normally this would not be such a comical scenario, but lately the blonde finds all of these little problems funny. I told him if he wanted to be tended to he should have gone to my parent's house, my mom is much better at nursing people back to health than me. So to tally up the score card . . . Lauren is on the mend, although I kept her home an extra day. J.J., still at my folks, will be picked up shortly, the husband is acting like a big whiney baby. Alicia and the mother are just fine. We will be spending the day at the mall just to get away from all these sickies!

I hope you are all well. If not . . . STAY AWAY!! LOL

Rene & Alicia

Subject: Alicia Update January 15
1/15/2003 10:46:04 AM Eastern Standard Time

One year ago today Alicia's Uncle John detected her spinal tumor and she was admitted to the hospital for surgery. It's amazing how these dates stick out in the blonde one's mind, when I can't remember what I did yesterday! Luckily, she is feeling just fine (it's amazing what some anti nausea medicine can do). It appears that she and I have dodged the "virus bullet" that everyone else had succumbed to in this house. I knew by yesterday morning that everyone was feeling just fine though when they all were charmingly cranky!

We went yesterday to pick out Alicia's Communion dress. God bless Nanny and Grandpa for their ability to "spoil" our little patient. Have to admit, this dress is prettier than my wedding dress, well at least on of them (long story, I had 2 . . . Dresses not weddings. You know there is always a "story" where I am concerned. LOL). Anyway, we will go for a fitting next week and hopefully we will be able to pick out a veil for our patient. The store is making up one to cover most of her head since she will probably have not much more than some fuzz at the time. It was an exciting day for Alicia as she tried on no less than 15 dresses. Have to admit, it felt positively wonderful to see her so happy!

Tonight is J.J.'s band concert. Alicia is already negotiating her way out of this. As she put it to me . . . "you know I'm on chemotherapy, and there could be sick people there." (The mother and she are going to have a hard time when we no longer have our chemotherapy excuse LOL). She is right though, and will probably stay with a neighbor.

Tomorrow is clinic and Friday morning Jingle Belle is going to the vet.

Hope everyone is staying warm!
Rene & Alicia

RENE A. FESLER

Subject: Alicia Update January 16
1/16/2003 5:22:58 PM Eastern Standard Time

Alicia went to clinic and sailed through her blood tests. She did so well, we don't even have to go back until her last admittance on Monday January 27th. YEAH!

Unfortunately, both my parents have been feeling a bit under the weather since their weekend infirmary for the kids. Fortunately, it hasn't been too bad for them, just a little queasy. Everyone in the Giacalone household is feeling just fine, except the mother who is very tired lately. (Guess life is catching up to me).

We did our standard lunch, and then needed to get home to check on Jingle Belle (my life is now ruled by a dog! LOL). Tomorrow she is going to the vet for the first time. Like I don't do enough doctors as it is! LOL

Hope everyone's weekend is great. Kids are off on Monday

Enjoy!
Rene & Alicia

Subject: Alicia Update January 21
1/21/2003 11:54:22 AM Eastern Standard Time

Hope everyone had a good weekend. Alicia's was filled with her typical sleepovers and partying with her friends. It's just a shame that youth is wasted on the young! She is feeling good, other than an occasional queasy stomach, but she has medication to help this.

Yesterday the kids enjoyed the day off with playing and a little shopping. Unfortunately, Jingle Belle got out of the yard again! This is starting to get old! The wind we experienced yesterday blew one of the fenced down in the yard. We sent her out, thinking she was in the yard, while she was enjoying herself running up and down the block. Luckily, Lauren found her while I re-attached the fence. (Woman with tool . . . watch out! LOL)

No clinic this week, but a dress fitting tomorrow for Alicia with some lunch and a possible trip to the mall.

This Sunday we'll be enjoying Super Bowl at our friend's house. There is some friendly competition with him rooting for Oakland, and me for Tampa Bay. (It's the Florida thing for me.) Should make for a great day and although I am not normally the competitive type, when it comes to some good old fashioned football and this particular neighbor, I just can't help myself!

Next Monday January 27th is Alicia's last chemotherapy cycle and admittance (#17)!!!! Even though it is an overnight stay, we are putting out an invitation to anyone who would like to visit Monday afternoon or evening. We are planning on making this last stay ONE BIG PARTY!!! If you can make it great, if you can't, not a problem, you can always visit her at home.

Be well and stay warm!
Rene & Alicia

Subject: Alicia Update January 27th
1/27/2003 3:56:51 PM Eastern Standard Time

Alicia is admitted and finally in her room. Unfortunately, right now her telephone isn't working and we are awaiting the arrival of the telephone repair man. Accessing went beautifully as the oncology nurses did their usual great job. We hung out in clinic for most of the day and just got to her room about 45 minutes ago. We JUST made our numbers to get chemo (could you imagine with all the excitement of the last time if we got sent home?) and chemo has yet to be hung. We are having a problem getting Alicia's tinkle to cooperate. We are trying to fit in a CAT scan and bone scan tomorrow and with the late hour that chemo is going to be hung today, looks like we might not be home till tomorrow evening sometime.

Getting Alicia up here today took a little bit of doing. She is feeling a little sad that her life as she has known it for the past year is about to change. She has made many friends up here and she keeps on questioning me if she'll be able to visit. I believe it is a normal reaction for anyone, even though personally I am just feeling relieved. We are presently awaiting the arrival of Lauren and J.J. with Grandpa.

Hope everyone is well.

How did you like that super Bowl? I won myself a case of White Castle . . . life IS good!

Rene & Alicia

WHAT MY FRIENDS HAVE LEARNED . . .

A T VARIOUS TIMES throughout Alicia's treatment, I would get e-mails from friends and family. Sometimes it was in direct response to a question or request of mine, other times it was just the few words of encouragement or support that someone felt compelled to write. As Alicia was nearing the end of her treatment, I received the following e-mail from a friend of mine. Someone who I had met through Alicia and whose friendship I value. She is not someone who I see often and actually don't even speak to her that much; however, through my year of e-mails, a friendship and bond was forged. I found in her words an understanding and new meaning as to the impact of Alicia's illness not only upon me, but upon those around me. While my e-mails were therapy for me to bare my soul and communicate the fears I lived with, they turned out to be, for many people, an invaluable lesson about life. I never wanted the world to view Alicia with pity or sorrow. I didn't want people whispering words of sorrow about the circumstances surrounding our family. I wanted people to look with wonder and amazement at the example of strength, perseverance, and courage that Alicia exemplified. I wanted me and my children to embrace life and enjoy it with all the zest that we could possibly muster. I wanted our suffering and fears to help others in their lives. The following words from my friend confirmed for me that this year of cancer care wasn't for naught, for as horrible and difficult it was for all of us, it gave many people a new appreciation of life.

Subject: Re: Alicia Update January 30
1/31/2003 6:31:26 AM Eastern Standard Time

Dear Rene & Alicia

It is with great joy and pride that I congratulate you both on the completion of treatment! You asked us all long ago to tell you what we learned from your experience of the past year, and after much soul searching I have come up with some things: I have learned there is nothing stronger than the power of a mother's love (even a blonde one)-I have learned that sheer will and determination can overcome-I have learned that true friends don't have to see each other often to have a deep connection-I have learned that the sun always comes up the next day, no matter how bad the previous day was-I have learned that tears don't ruin a computer's keyboard-I have learned that families can grow stronger in the face of adversity-I have learned that community support can come when you least expect it-I have learned to appreciate every day-I have learned that good can overcome evil-I have learned that joy can be found even in sorrow-I have learned that my friend Rene is a fantastic writer (I am an English Teacher, sorry)-I have learned what true courage is and it is a beautiful little girl named ALICIA. Let's all celebrate ALICIA!

Love,
Shari

Subject: Alicia Update February 5
2/4/2003 8:17:03 PM Eastern Standard Time

Alicia had her first clinic visit today as a "cancer-survivor" post chemo. She did "marvelously." In fact she did so well that she is now done with her Neupogen shots (white count) and should only have two more weeks of her Aranesp (red count). The mother is more than happy to give up the role of nurse. We do not have to go back for 3 weeks which will be the week after our Florida vacation; and it is a well deserved vacation I might add. Alicia also had an echocardiogram this morning which looked just fine. We just need to complete an MRI and CAT scan next Tuesday and then we get to veg for a little while. Life is good in the Giacalone household.

Now to give everyone a little chuckle at the "blonde one's" expense (I still have my sense of humor) it appears I have finally met my match. I have run up against someone who is totally unphased and unaffected by me. Any requests or directions I give are met with indifference and non-compliance. Any attempts I make to control a situation are totally disregarded. I am at a loss . . . to a 4 pound puppy named Jingle Belle! Nothing is quite as frustrating as this little thing just wagging her tail, running around the neighborhood and charging her little body into the gates to knock them down. And all the while . . . I'm just wondering "how the hell did I handle cancer, yet I can't handle this dog?" She keeps me humble and frustrated to say the least! LOL

There is an upcoming cocktail party for the Children's Cancer Center and Honeysuckle Foundation on Thursday May 15. Any of you interested in attending this event, please email me your address so an invitation can be sent. Yes, I will be attending. Wouldn't miss any opportunity to have fun!

Everyone be well!
Rene & Alicia

Subject: Alicia Update February 11
Date 2/11/03 5:24:10 PM Eastern Standard Time

Alicia is doing great. We went today to complete her CAT scan and MRI at her Uncle John's office in Brooklyn and I am pleased to inform everyone . . . things look great! (The most exciting part of the day was viewing the cookies and milk she had just eaten that were now in her tummy LOL).

Things have settled down into a more "normal" pattern with a snow day last Friday and our upcoming Florida vacation with friends of ours next week. It has been over a year since we have been down south, and the anticipation and excitement have gripped the Giacalone household. (I don't know who's more excited the kids or the mother?)

Lauren and J.J. are doing well and the dog . . . well, the dog is the dog. Not going to let the four pound fur ball get to me. She's going to spend all of next week at my parents house . . . let her get to them! LOL

Wednesday J.J. and Alicia's school is hosting a cupcake sale as a fundraiser for our Foundation, so tonight we will be baking. Alicia has packed already. J.J. is finishing up the last of hockey and 6 AM Saturday morning its "Naples . . . here we come!!!!!!"

Hope everyone is well and enjoys next week!

Gee, it feels kind of strange not going to the hospital for a change . . . NOT!!!! I do miss all of our North Shore friends though!

Love
Rene & Alicia

Subject: Alicia Update February 17
Date: 2/17/03 8:26:27 PM Eastern Standard Time

We are in Naples and enjoying ourselves immensely! Sorry for all the snow the northerners are dealing with . . . NOT! LOL I'm just glad we missed it. Thank you fellow Honeysucklians for keeping my driveway clear.

Weather is spectacular, water is warm, food and drink delicious and the company is wonderful. Alicia is especially enjoying some time as a regular kid. Although it felt like it never would come, it sure feels good coming home. Planned for the next few days are fishing, boating, shelling, shopping, going to the beach and all around partying!

Life is wonderful!

Love
Rene & Alicia

Last I heard New York had about 20 inches of snow . . . is that correct? LOL

Subject: Alicia Update February 19
Date 2/19/03 3:58:01 PM Eastern Standard Time

Well the Giacalone's never can do anything without a story. This sage began on Tuesday when our friend's daughter came down with a fever. Today she is feeling better, but unfortunately who should come down with a fever . . . Alicia. (Do NOT worry North Shore friends; the mother has it under control.☺) There is nothing that we can't handle. Needless to say, we have had a rotation of parents staying with sick kids. Good thing we are home and not at a hotel, otherwise it would be a pain. Still, rather be in Naples with fever than in New York with ALL that snow.

Other than that minor speed bump, we are all having a great time. What could be bad wearing shorts, looking at palm trees and sipping on Pina Coladas? Not a damn thing!

Hope everyone up north is enjoying their time off if they have it. Barring any weather problems or icing problems in Cincinnati (that's where we stopover and we had that coming down), we should be landing sometime Sunday evening around 9PM. School on Monday is negotiable, since I might be too tired to wake everyone up! LOL.

Be well and warm!
Rene & Alicia

Subject: Honeysuckle Foundation for Children with Cancer
Date: 2/24/03 1:00:13 Eastern Standard Time

I don't know if I have mentioned it before, but on Thursday May 15, North Shore Pediatric Cancer Center along with our Foundation will be hosting a cocktail party, silent auction at the Metropolitan in Glen Cove. We are looking for donations for the silent auction and I am putting out a call to any and everyone who might be able to secure any donations. I have letters in my possession explaining the event and will be more than happy to send them to anyone who would require them. If you don't have a connection, maybe you have a friend or relative who does and would be able to assist. If you would like to attend this event (I hope all my friends do LOL) please send me your address and the addresses of any friends of yours who might also like to attend.

Thank you and have a nice day!

Rene & Alicia

Subject: Alicia Update February 28
Date: 2/28/03 11:35:25 AM Eastern Standard Time

Alicia went to clinic this week and did fine. She needed to have her mediport accessed to make sure it is clear, but in usual Alicia style it was not a problem. Her white count was a little low, but her other numbers were good and we don't have to go back for a month. (Not that we won't miss all of you, we now just pop in for social visits!) She has been very tired this week and naps everyday. (I am feeling quite drained myself this week, I wonder why?)

I've attached some vacation photos. Of course there is always a story when we're involved . . . eating dinner at one of the resorts on the beach one evening (you have to sip cocktails while watching the sunset) water suddenly came pouring down from one of the upper floors. Seems there was a sprinkler malfunction. Of course the fire department needs to check it out, (check out these firemen!!!) And we had to stop and take pictures of course.

Another day some bird of prey (looked like an eagle to me) scooped a catfish out of the lake and ate it on the shore. After that . . . vultures, at least a dozen of them were circling overhead. (I had to admit, I thought they were looking for me! LOL)

We also just had some good old fun sunning, swimming and going out to dinner.

Hope everyone enjoys their weekend. We will be guests of the Islanders (thank you Ms. Rosemary) tomorrow evening in their luxury skybox. You know it's tough being social, but someone has to do it! LOL.

Be well
Rene & Alicia

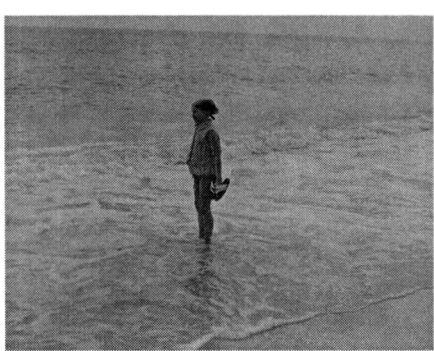 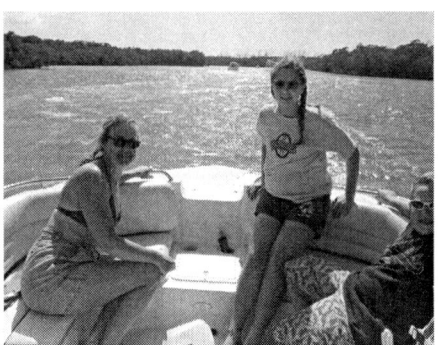

Subject: Alicia Update March 12
Date: 3/12/03 11:57:19 AM Eastern Standard Time

Well I am happy to report that is Alicia is doing just fine. She has "fuzz" on her head, along with eyebrows and eyelashes. (I never thought I would be so excited over this.) In fact she is doing so well; she went to school today as a "visitor." We might as well try to get her back into the routine. Other than being tired (aren't we all LOL) she is actually feeling quite good. Now what shall the mother do with herself with all that free time? She's been home with me since December 2001 . . . gee time flies when you're having fun!

Last weekend we "launched" the spring season (hey we're anxious, this winter has been tooooo long) with a bar-b-cue on the blocks new "fire pit." It is the suburban version of a 50 gallon drum in the middle of the street. LOL. A little snow on the ground could never stop us . . . we just like to have fun. Monday evening we were visited by "Make A Wish Foundation." Alicia wants to go on a 7 day Disney cruise, which they are now working on. She is officially a "wish kid." Finishing up with J.J.'s hockey and preparing for all the end of school year activities including Lauren's confirmation and graduation, J.J.'s graduation and Alicia's First Holy Communion. All good stuff for a change! Life is wonderful!

Those of you who have pledged items for the silent auction/cocktail party . . . thank you so much for your support. Anyone with any connections that would like to donate anything (ex. Gift certificates to restaurants, spas, stores or any items) . . . we would truly appreciate any help we get. Be on the lookout for your invitations, they will be arriving shortly.

Still haven't locked in our golf date, a friend of mine is tirelessly working on this project for us.

Keep smiling and everyone be well!

Rene & Alicia (who's at school)

Subject: Alicia Update March 13
Date: 3/13/03 2:05:35 PM Eastern Standard Time

Alicia stayed in school yesterday for the bulk of the day and went again this morning. Unfortunately, the mother got a call while at Costco by 10:30 AM to pick her up. Yesterday she was operating on pure adrenaline and today it caught up to her. She was excited to see her friends and sit at her desk. She said everyone was asking her how she was feeling and then said, "Do you think anybody knows I had cancer? I didn't want to say anything because I didn't want anybody to feel bad for me," out of the mouths of babes.

The mother is just as glad she is home today. Yesterday, Jingle Belle got out of the yard . . . again. Do you think she knew I was on my own and would be trotting up and down the block myself? LOL Well that didn't happen, I found her down the block, opened up the door and waited for her to come in. Unfortunately, I couldn't get her out from under the bed, but at least she was in the house.

Tonight we will be going to the elementary school for Curriculum Night to see some of J.J. and Alicia's work. Tomorrow is Friday and another weekend is here! We do LOVE the weekends!

Regarding the question some of you have asked, can you pay at the door for the cocktail party? Yes you can. However, if you pay in advance (VISA/MC/ AMEX) you avoid waiting on line that evening and can get right to the cocktail party and silent auction. You know I WILL be pre-registered. Details will be forthcoming.

Have a great day!
Rene & Alicia

Subject: Wisdom
Date: 3/15/03 8:57:33 AM Eastern Standard Time

Although this is supposedly for women only, I think there are some valuable lessons here for everyone.

Enjoy!

Let's wear purple hats!
In honor of women's history month and in memory of Erma Bombeck who lost her fight with cancer. Here is an angel sent over to watch over you. Pass this on to five women that you want watched over. If you don't know five women to pass this on to, one will do just fine.

IF I HAD MY LIFE TO LIVE OVER

By Erma Bombeck
(Written after she found out she was dying from cancer)

I would have gone to bed when I was sick instead of pretending the earth would go into a holding pattern if I weren't there for a day.

I would have burned the pink candle sculpted like a rose before it melted in storage.

I would have talked less and listened more.

I would have invited friends over to dinner even if the carpet was stained, or the sofa was faded.

I would have eaten the popcorn in the "good" living room and worried much less about the dirt when someone wanted to light a fire in the fireplace.

RENE A. FESLER

I would have taken more time to listen to my grandfather ramble about his youth.

I would never have insisted the car windows be rolled up on a summer day because my hair had just been teased and sprayed . . .

I would have sat on the lawn with my grass stains.

I would have cried and laughed less while watching television and more while watching life.

I would never have bought anything just because it was practical, wouldn't show soil, or was guaranteed to last a lifetime.

Instead of wishing away nine months of pregnancy, I'd have cherished every moment and realized that the wonderment growing inside me was the only chance in life to assist God in a miracle.

When my kids kissed me impetuously, I would never have said, "later. Now go get washed up for dinner." There would have been more "I love you's." More 'I'm sorry's."

But most importantly, given another shot at life, I would seize every minute . . . look at it and really see it . . . live it . . . and never give it back. Stop sweating the small stuff.

Don't worry about who doesn't like you, who has more, or who's doing what.

Instead, let's cherish the relationships we have with those who do love us.

Let's think about what God HAS blessed us with. And what we are doing each day to promote ourselves mentally, physically, emotionally. We have one shot at life and then it's gone. I hope you all have a blessed day.

Beautiful Women's Month

> *Age 3: She looks at herself and sees a Queen*
> *Age 8: She looks at herself and sees Cinderella*
> *Age 15: She looks at herself and sees an Ugly Sister (Mom I can't go to school looking like this!)*

Age 20: *She looks at herself and sees 'too fat/too thin, too short/too tall, and too straight/too curly:-but decides she's going out anyway.*

Age 30: *She looks at herself at herself and sees "too fat/too thin, too short/ too tall, too straight/too curly," but decides she doesn't have time to fix it, so she's going out anyway.*

Age 40: *She looks at herself and sees "clean" and goes out anyway.*

Age 50: *She looks at herself and sees "I am" and goes wherever she wants to go.*

Age 60: *She looks at herself and reminds herself of all the people who can't even see themselves in the mirror anymore. Goes out and conquers the world.*

Age 70: *She looks at herself and sees wisdom, laughter, and ability, goes out and enjoys life.*

Age 80: *Doesn't bother to look. Just puts on a purple hat and goes out to have fun in the world.*

Send this on to all the women you are grateful to have as friends. Maybe we should all grab that purple hat earlier. Please send this to five phenomenal women today in celebration of Beautiful Women's Month. If you do, something good will happen: you will boost another woman's self esteem.

Even if you're on the right track, you'll get run over if you just sit there—Will Rogers

Subject: Alicia Update March 18
Date: 3/18/03 1:55:42 PM Eastern Standard Time

Alicia has been doing well. She goes into school and comes home around lunch time. She is not use to a schedule and tires quite easily. She is trying however, and that is all anyone can ask for.

The weather has been glorious the past few days (it's about time) and I think everyone is happy to see winter leave.

I want to share something with everyone that I hope you will see some relevance in. As many of you are aware, the past year, since 9/11 has been very challenging for us as with many people. The loss of a family friend on 9/11, then Alicia's cancer, the loss of

Alicia's friend Sarah, the trauma just seems never ending. Within the past 2 weeks, 2 of our neighbors have both lost their mothers. While one was sickly and older, the other was a 63 year old vibrant woman who had a terrible accident. Both were tragic, in that nobody is ever prepared to say "goodbye," and loss is hurt no matter what age or what the circumstances. Lauren and I attended the funeral today and I have to admit, I found it easier to get through Alicia's cancer care than to comfort someone else. It is only recently that I truly could appreciate what all of you felt when Alicia was diagnosed. I was at a loss for words (I know hard to imagine). So today I embraced my friend, whose grief was overwhelming, and offered my prayers and condolences and any assistance she or her family may need. Trivial some may say, but very much needed by everyone from time to time . . . which leads me to my point (yes this rambling is going somewhere, work with me I am on a roll!) With the impending war and gloom and doom wherever we turn lately, let's each and every one of us try to do something "good" for those who are truly important in our lives. Let's not wait for there to be a reason like cancer or death. (No, I am not saying turn into a Pollyanna. That isn't my style! LOL). Make a phone call; send a letter drop over with a cake. Let someone know just how important they are to you . . . go out of your comfort zone and make a difference somewhere to someone who might not otherwise know it. It may seem corny or ridiculous, but little acts of kindness mean more than you will ever know and in light of everything going on . . . we need this NOW! All those "little trivial things" that so many of you did for us, made a huge difference when we were struggling with Alicia's cancer. The basis for our Foundation was all the concern and kindness exhibited by all of you. Make something positive where there otherwise might not be any. People deserve it . . . and we deserve it ourselves!

I will now put my puka beads away, fold up my meditation mat and snuff out the incense! LOLOL.

Be well
Rene & Alicia

Subject: Alicia's Communion Date
Date: 3/19/03 4:21:22 PM Eastern Standard Time

Please pencil in the date . . . Alicia's First Holy Communion
Saturday May 24th at the 9:00 AM Mass
Details and invitations will be forthcoming

Subject: Alicia Update March 24
Date: 3/24/03 3:38:15 PM Eastern Standard Time

Hope this email finds everyone well. March is moving right along and the arrival of spring has made the kids happy along with some adults I know. It is quite reassuring seeing all the kids on their bicycles and running up and down the block. Especially with the current war situation it makes me think that no matter how dismal or dark things might get, there will always be a bright sunny day just around the corner.

Alicia is feeling just fine and is due back at clinic next week: April 1st. (Antonella that is correct, right?) She goes into school whenever she can and is gradually building up her stamina. I am happy to report that both Alicia and Lauren along with a friend tried out for a play at a local community theater and they both made it. Now we will have two divas in training, like they weren't high maintenance already? Oh those high maintenance women, I just can't deal with them! LOL

Let me catch you up to date with Jingle Belle. The story now sounds better than the actual event . . . I have to admit, I thought she was a goner! She got out of the yard yesterday and almost ran out of the development. If it wasn't for a lady in her car stopping and jumping out, she would have headed straight out onto the main road. All my friends and I, after frantically chasing her, spent yesterday securing the yard to prevent her escape . . . so what should happen today? She got out again with Alicia and I home . . . missed getting hit by a SUV by only a few feet . . . and had me and Alicia, who was hysterically crying, and a workman working in the development who joined us in the chase, running all over the neighborhood. Thank goodness we caught her and she is now tethered to a puppy stake in the yard, or is in the house under "house arrest." The unpredictability of this dog could have cost her her life, and there was absolutely nothing I could do about it. Just another example that no matter how much we believe we have "control" over our lives and our destiny, we don't. Other than our own actions, we are totally vulnerable to the acts of others, even 5 pound dogs!

Be well
Rene & Alicia

PS. Mark your calendars for the cocktail party, Thursday May 15th!

RENE A. FESLER

Subject: Foundation Information
Date: 3/25/03 3:50:43 PM Eastern Standard Time

I'm sure you're surprised to hear from me so soon (aren't you all so lucky LOL) but I do need to address some things regarding the Foundation that many of you have inquired about.

First, we have NOT sent any invitations out yet for the cocktail party (Thursday May 15th @ the Metropolitan in Glen Cove) . . . we are working on it. Hey, I'm trying to figure out this computer stuff. Although I have many of your addresses, if you think I might not, please email it to me, along with the names and addresses of any other people you might want invited, the more the merrier. There will be a RSVP card along with instructions on how to pre-register, which will save you standing on line the night of the affair (more time for cocktails and bidding!)

Second ANYONE can make a donation to the silent auction. (Thank you to those who already have). It doesn't have to be a business or organization. A wonderful suggestion is a gift certificate. Anyone making a donation can send them directly to me along with the names and address of the donor, so proper credit can be given. If you need to have your donation picked up, let me know and I will make arrangements.

Thirdly, I do not have the date for the golf outing yet. We are working on it, and as soon as we have that information, I will be forwarding it to all of you.

That is all for now, I look forward to seeing you all very soon!

Rene

Subject: Hugs for Sarah
Date: 3/30/03 3:55:21 PM Eastern Standard Time

I remember Sarah's birthday last year as though it was yesterday. It was Easter Sunday and the goal was to get her out of the hospital to celebrate at home. What a year this has been, to think she is not even here to celebrate this one, is beyond comprehension. Who would believe that such a thing was possible? I know as a parent having a child diagnosed with cancer, the diagnosis itself seemed horrific enough, let alone her death. Unfortunately, it is all too real and something that should bring us all back to reality.

I've said it before and I'll say it again . . . each one of us has a gift; our life and the blessing of those around us! Don't sweat the small stuff, keep things in their proper perspective, don't just coast through life, make a difference and make things happen! The most difficult thing for anyone to do is to go out of our own "comfort zone" (that area we feel most content in) and push the envelope. We are all capable of great things, look no further than the valiant fight these "cancer kids" put up! Are the stresses and problems we have more difficult than anything these children are faced with? Are you able to channel your energy for the benefit of your friends and loved ones and more importantly yourself? Remember, self-respect and strong self-worth is key to facing anything that comes your way. I am not the person I was prior to Alicia's diagnosis. I am not even the same person I was prior to Sarah's death. I have little patience for minutia and those who get bogged down in it along with their negative energy. I do however, realize how much we need one another. Our family and friends make it all seem worthwhile and help us get through ANYTHING! We can never know the suffering felt by Sarah's family, as you will never know the heartache endured by my family. What I do know though, is not a day goes by that I don't pause for a moment to reflect on what we have gone through, where we hope to go and then try to do something about it. My life plan has taken on a whole new meaning and direction. Each of you has that same opportunity without experiencing our grief, so what are you waiting for?

Hugs & Kisses
Rene & Alicia

Subject: Alicia Update April 3
Date: 4/3/03 5:11:38 PM Eastern Standard Time

Hope this email finds everyone happy and healthy . . . everyone in our household is holding their own. The kids are excited to be outside and I already planted some perennials . . . last year's neglect has caught up to my garden LOL.

Alicia went to clinic on Monday for her monthly check up and port accessing; her numbers are good and she has put on three pounds. She was wonderful with the accessing and enjoys her new status as strictly a "visitor." We visited the pediatric floor and then got to go home. We do not miss staying up on the seventh floor for one minute! Originally, we were planning on having her mediport removed six months from the end of chemotherapy. After some discussion with her doctor however, we decided to leave it in for a year. It

RENE A. FESLER

hasn't given her any trouble, and it is just easier for testing to do an access versus an IV. (Alicia would much rather have the port accessed than an IV anyway!) We will go back again the beginning of May, what was the date and time Antonella? The pediatric oncology department has implemented stricter rules for visits and admissions. You now have to go at an appointed time. They told me they waited for Alicia to finish treatment before they started this, since they felt I wouldn't "abide" by the new rules. Where the heck do you think they got that impression from? LOL.

Check your mail; you should be receiving that invitation for the cocktail party by the end of the weekend. If you don't get one, let me know and I'll make sure you do. Still looking for any donations, and hopefully I will be able to send you a "save the date" email for our golf outing which is tentatively looking like July 21st (J.J.'s birthday). I will let you know however as soon as it is firmed up.

Stay well and be happy!
Rene & Alicia

PS: Antonella, see I didn't make you cry today!!!!!

Subject: Save the date!
Date: 4/10/03 10:43:25 AM Eastern Daylight Time

I am happy to announce, we have secured the Hempstead Golf and Country Club on Monday July 21, 2003 at 12:30 for our First Annual Honeysuckle Foundation for Children with Cancer Golf Classic. Please mark your calendars. I will be looking for assistance from anyone and everyone who wants to help. If you have friends, relatives, work colleagues or business associates who would like to attend this event or be a sponsor, please email me their addresses and phone numbers.

When I have more details, I will forward them to all of you. In the meantime, if you could all start assembling the names and addresses for our invitation list, I will be very much indebted . . . (And it will prevent me from harassing the heck out of you LOLOLOL!) I'm kidding, just because I've gone legit doesn't mean I've lost my sense of humor!

Rene

Subject: Alicia Update April 20
Date: 4/20/03 11:28:45 PM Eastern Daylight Time

I hope this email finds everyone well . . . a little stuffed from all the holiday feasting I'm sure. Alicia has been feeling just fine although she still is unable to go into McDonald's (it makes her extremely nauseous), but J.J. is working on that. Being off this week with the kids should be fun, although it looks like they are booking up their time real fast.

We did Honeysuckle Court egg decorating in front of our house yesterday, an Easter egg hunt up and down the block this afternoon, and an evening hunt for the adults. Yes Shannon, we are just like the "Truman Show" LOL.

Alicia was excited about the arrival of the Easter bunny . . . let's face it, after the years of innocence she has lost due to cancer, we are holding onto childhood as long as we can. I sometimes forget just how "deep" and pensive she can be and once again has proved what an incredibly compassionate human being she is. A friend of ours is expecting a baby in May. Unfortunately, during a routine sonogram a problem was detected with the baby's heart. The baby will need open heart surgery 2 days after her birth, her prognosis is excellent, but awaiting her birth is bittersweet. Something that should be a wonderfully joyous event will be met with fear and stress. I know this family will handle everything with strength and perseverance, as they are strong people. I have said on one or two occasions that God only gives you what you can handle! I had to tell my kids about this and of course they are all upset. Saturday evening after everyone went to bed, it seems a little cancer survivor tiptoed downstairs to leave a personal message to the Easter bunny. (Antonella get your tissues ready).

Dear Easter Bunny,

I love you. Happy Easter! I have a friend and her mom is having a baby and the baby needs an operation because it has a heart thing so pray for the baby PLEASE!

I want a few things . . . I want a new game boy and games for the game boy.
(This is the part she takes after her mother LOL)

Love
Alicia

As the MasterCard commercial says "Priceless!"

I know firsthand what the power of prayer and positive energy are capable of doing, so I am asking you all to pray for our friends and their unborn daughter.

Every good thought and prayer helps!

Take Care
Rene & Alicia

Subject: Alicia Update April 26
Date: 4/27/03 8:48:40 AM Eastern Daylight Time

I hope this email finds everyone well . . . hard to believe that spring break is over. They say that time flies when you are having fun . . . guess we must be having a blast! We did a trip to Manhattan on the Long Island Railroad with the girls, and visited my brother at his company offices. We went to Six Flags Great Adventure in New Jersey on a whim and J.J. had a visit to the auto show in New York City.

Easter was a lot of fun with an Easter egg hunt for the kids and then a "twilight" hunt for the parents . . . too much candy though.

Alicia has been thoroughly enjoying herself, being a "fish" in the "Little Mermaid" every weekend and playing soccer. She does tire, but with the schedule we've been keeping lately, even I am a little tuckered out!

Foundation business has been keeping me very busy, all good stuff I might add, and I am looking forward to all the upcoming fundraising activities. Our website is under construction, but if you go to the site you can see our logo.

www.honeysucklefoundation.org
If you email something to the Foundation, it comes to me. I don't know how, but I think it is cool. Our webmaster has been working feverishly on the site for us, we are very lucky to have him on our team.

We will probably be going to clinic soon . . . Antonella, could you check for me? And we are taking it just one day at a time.

Be Well
Rene & Alicia

Thought you all might find this inspirational!

Great Food for Thought

Michael is the kind of guy you love to hate.

He is always in a good mood and always has something positive to say.

When someone would ask him how he was doing, he would reply, "If I were any better I would be twins!" He was a natural motivator. If an employee was having a bad day, Michael was there telling the employee to look on the positive side of the situation.

Seeing this style made me curious, so one day I went up to Michael and asked him, "I don't get it! You can't be a positive person all of the time. How do you do it?"

Michael replied, "Each morning I wake up and say to myself, you have two choices today. You can choose to be in a good mood, or you can choose to be in a bad mood. I choose to be in a good mood. Each time something bad happens, I can choose to be a victim or I can choose to learn from it. I choose to learn from it. Every time someone comes to me complaining, I can choose to accept their complaining or I can point out the positive side of life. I choose the positive side of life."

"Yeah right, it's not that easy," I protested. "Yes it is" Michael said. "Life is all about choices. When you cut away all the junk, every situation is a choice.

You choose how you react to situations.

You choose how people affect your moods

You choose to be in a good mood or a bad mood.

The bottom line: It's your choice how to live your life."

I reflected on what Michael said. Soon thereafter, I left the Tower industry to start my own business. Michael and I lost touch, but I often thought about him when I made a choice about life instead of just reacting to it.

Several years later, I heard that Michael was involved in a serious accident, falling some 60 feet from a communication tower. After 18 hours of surgery and weeks of intensive care, Michael was released from the hospital with rods placed in his back. I saw Michael about six months after the accident. When I asked him how he was, he replied, "If I were any better, I'd be twins. Want to see my scars?"

I declined to see his wounds, but I did ask him what had gone through his mind as the accident took place. "The first thing that went through my mind was the well-being of my soon to be born daughter." Michael replied. "Then as I lay on the ground, I remembered I had two choices: I could choose to live or I could choose to die. I chose to live."

"Weren't you scared? Did you lose consciousness?" I asked.

Michael continued, "The paramedics were great. They kept telling me I was going to be fine, but when they wheeled me into the ER and I saw the expressions on the faces of the doctors and nurses, I got really scared. In their eyes, I read 'he's a dead man.' I knew I needed to take action."

"What did you do?" I asked. "Well, there was a big burly nurse shouting questions at me," said Michael. "She asked if I was allergic to anything. "Yes I replied." The doctors and nurses stopped working at they waited for my reply. I took a deep breath and yelled, "Gravity." Over their laughter I told them, "I am choosing to live. Operate on me as if I am alive, not dead."

Attitude, after all, is everything. "Therefore do not worry about tomorrow, for tomorrow will worry about itself. Each day has enough trouble of its own. After all today is the tomorrow you worried about yesterday."

You have two choices now.

1. Delete this.
2. Forward it to the people you care about.

You know the choice I made.

Enjoy each day, each breath and mostly each and every friend.

Subject: Alicia Update May 6
Date: 5/6/03 10:15:47 AM Eastern Daylight Time

Good morning everyone! Hope this email finds you all well on a rainy cold day in New York. There is sunshine however, I am happy to report that our friends had their little baby girl this morning. She was close to 8 pounds, pink and crying. God Bless her. She is scheduled for heart surgery Friday morning, so let's get our prayer circle going and send lots of love and positive energy their way . . . look what your energy did for us!

Alicia is doing great! We were supposed to go to clinic this morning and the patient started to cry when she realized she had a field trip to go on . . . not a problem . . . we'll just go tomorrow. Thanks all my nursing friends for being so flexible! It's interesting how just 6 months ago, not a thought would have been given to the school activity . . . that was not Alicia's reality, the hospital was. What a wonderful problem to have wanting to be part of a field trip, school and being with her friends!

We started sending out the invitations for our golf outing so check your mail. I realize this is a pricey event and I know that I cannot expect everyone to attend. What I hope to accomplish with our Foundation is the ability for people to do as much or as little as they choose to do. (I like some form of involvement better than none LOL). Let's face it; fundraising is a luxury item these days. So when your invitation arrives and you just can't do this event, don't feel bad and don't throw the invitation out. What I would like and am asking you to do is to pass it on to your friends who might possibly join us. I need your contacts, since I have none of my own! I need to reach out beyond our inner circle to all of your inner circles. Whether it's your work associates, employer, family or your friends, we NEED to expand our network. That is the only way we will succeed! We have an idea floating around right now about raffling off a car at the golf outing, possibly a Mercedes Benz. If we can make this happen we would need to sell 800 tickets for $100 a piece. Would you go to your circle and sell them for us? What kind of commitment can I expect from each of you? I would love to hear from all of you about this . . . even if its just to say you couldn't do anything (at least I would then know you still read these emails LOL), I need your input! The blonde is treading new waters and needs all of you for help.

Please email me back with your thoughts . . .

Thanks again to all of you who are participating in our cocktail party next Thursday night. We had a meeting last night and I saw the final prize list. There are some absolutely wonderful prizes . . . and enough that there is something for everyone! If you are planning to attend and haven't sent in your registration yet, you must do so. There will be "special" raffles for those who are pre-registered and you might as well make yourselves eligible for some incredible additional prizes by sending your check in now!

We will have a great time and I look forward to having a cocktail with all of you! LOL

Be well
Rene, home alone . . . that's a good thing!

Subject: WEBSITE OPEN!
Date: 5/7/03 3:42:29 PM Eastern Daylight Time

It is with much pride and joy I announce the grand-opening of the Honeysuckle Foundation for Children with Cancer website which was generously donated to the Foundation from one of our Board Members Jason of WWWEBTEK (anyone needing web design and development, he's the man!) Hip, hip, hooray!!!! (We are still working out some typos and bugs!)

www.honeysucklefoundation.org
Please visit it and pass it along to all of your friends!

Thanks
Rene

Let me know what you think!

Subject: Alicia Update May 13
Date: 5/13/03 2:01:05 PM Eastern Daylight Time

Hope this email finds everyone well and that all mom's enjoyed their Mothers Day! Alicia is doing great, attending school everyday and playing with her friends. WE went to clinic last week and she did just fine. Actually we are due for another series of scans and tests . . . three months are up . . . time flies when you are having fun LOL. Let's hope there is nothing to "see" on these tests.

I want to thank everyone planning on attending Thursday night's cocktail party . . . I look forward to having a drink with all of you and doing a little "catching up." If you haven't sent in your check and would like to attend, please feel free to bring it along. They take checks and credit cards at the door. (I am starting to sound like an infomercial LOL) It is going to be a fun night!

Our invitations for the golf outing have been mailed and hopefully we will sell out soon . . . I am the eternal optimist! If you didn't receive one, or need more, let me know so I can get them to you pronto! I am putting out a plea for a volunteer donations/ raffle coordinator. The job description for this position is first you must be extremely organized (this discounted me!). You will be the contact person for all donations. You will be sending out letters to companies, sports teams, restaurants, stores, etc . . . . to secure donations. We will provide you with the letters, envelopes and postage. Then once you secure a donation, you will be in charge of the thank you letter sent to them. Again, this will be provided to you. This is truly an administrative type of position. We also need volunteers to "hit the streets" with letters in hand visiting any and all businesses to secure donations. Smaller businesses do better with a face and a name handing over a letter. We will provide you with the letters and will assist in picking up any donations you may get. I only ask you for your energy, time and any contact you may have. Even if it is just a friend, neighbor or relative every little bit helps and I need you! I am happy to report we got our first gift donation for the golf outing, 2 gift certificates to a local steak house. Actually, that's a gift I would like to win!

For all who have visited our website, thank you! I hope all of your will register and will become active visitors to this site. It will be an ever evolving project as we start to grow and you will not want to miss any of it!

For now, be well!

See you on Thursday
Rene & Alicia

Subject: Thank You!
Date: 5/16/03 11:42:12 AM Eastern Daylight Time

I would like to thank everybody who attended last night's cocktail party/silent auction. It was a great night and in my mind a huge success for our first fundraiser. I heard the food was excellent, I really didn't have much opportunity to eat (some may say my mouth was too busy talking to do any eating LOL). I am truly blessed to be surrounded by such an incredible group of caring people. You just prove it to me time and time again how genuinely special you all are!

Thanks Again!
Rene

Subject: Alicia Update May 19
Date: 5/19/03 10:22:36 AM Eastern Daylight Time

Just a quick update on what has been happening around here. Alicia has been feeling fine. A little bit of leg pain some evenings, but hopefully nothing to worry about since we don't want to get crazy. The weekend flew by as usual. Saturday was the last performance of the Little Mermaid, so my fish and mermaid are now "officially" retired for the summer season. We had a Communion party in New Jersey for a friend on Sunday and were lucky enough to spend more time in the car than at the party! (Alicia wanted to know if were driving to Florida LOL) I got to speak to some people at the party about the Foundation and people seemed very interested, especially in golf.

Stay well and try to stay warm . . . we are patiently awaiting the arrival of warm weather.

Rene & Alicia

Subject: Visit our Website!
Date: 5/20/03 9:39:27 AM Eastern Daylight Time

I want to let everyone know that you can now visit our website www.honeysucklefoundation. org and see photos of the cocktail party fundraiser. I think they all look great! If you haven't done so yet, please join our message board forums and post some messages, comments, questions, etc . . . .

Also, we are looking for a company to be our "shirt sponsor" for the golf outing and possibly donate shirts or fund the cost of them. Anybody work for a company or knows someone who does who might be able to help us out with this? Let us know, we probably need between 150-200 shirts. It's a great way for a company to get some good PR while helping out a worthy cause!

I look forward to hearing from all of you!

Enjoy your day!
Rene

Subject: Alicia Update May 26
Date: 5/26/03 10:54:07 AM Eastern Daylight Time

Happy Memorial Day to everyone! Although we think of this holiday as the "unofficial" start to the summer season, let's not forget those who have lost their lives enabling us to enjoy the freedom and lifestyle we all are fortunate to have. The weather has not been exactly cooperative this weekend though, so today I think I will start building me an ark! LOL Rain however, could not and did not dampen our spirits as we celebrated Alicia's First Holy Communion on Saturday. Yes, it has been a weekend event for us! We even had some people make it over from New Jersey for that early morning mass in weather that was anything other than ideal. Not that I am biased, but she looked spectacular and enjoyed herself immensely. Her receiving this sacrament for the first time had some people crying, and then her enjoyment at her party and the entire day brought more tears of joy and happiness. The party of course then moved onto Honeysuckle Court where the festivities continue even today. Saturday night was at our house and the party then moved about the block where there have been lacrosse games, sleepovers, painting parties and loads of food and drink and even some late night telephone calls to arouse partygoers from their beds. (I was not so appreciative when I received one of these calls, so I returned to the party in my PJ's!)

We are at the three month mark again as far as testing for Alicia. While I was planning on doing these tests within the next 2 weeks, Alicia was not feeling too good last week with some pain in her legs and her ribs. We made a quick change in plans and had a bone scan on Thursday, which I am pleased to say, showed absolutely nothing. We will do her CAT scan and MRI sometime this week and hopefully they will show us nothing also! The anxiety of pain however, had us all a bit on edge.

Next Saturday Lauren receives her Confirmation and then I have Lauren and J.J. both graduating. I cannot believe this; I am too young to have a daughter going into high school LOL. Although we are very busy the next 2 months, these are all wonderful things and I am just thankful we are all able to enjoy these together.

Quick golf updates, if you are planning on attending, please get your checks in soon. Looks like we are close to selling out! Yeah!!! Remember, if you don't golf, you can join us for the dinner portion. WE are still looking for dinner sponsorships and silent auction items. If you need some letters asking for these donations, please let me know and I will get them to you.

Be well and stay dry!
Rene & Alicia

Subject: Alicia Update June 2
Date: 6/2/03 4:16:58 PM Eastern Daylight Time

Another action packed weekend for everyone here as Lauren made her Confirmation on Saturday. We did lunch and Saturday night Alicia had a friend's birthday party at the Lady Rider's soccer game. (Yes it was outside in all that rain as I was an assistant driver). We got a wee bit wet, but the kids had a lot of fun and that's all that matters. Sunday we had a Bat Mitzvah for one of the oncology nurses daughters (you know our philosophy of once a friend of the blonde, always a friend of the blonde LOL) and today we are back to the grind. I wish I could have spent the whole day in bed!!!

Alicia is doing great and this week is filled with lots of "stuff." I wanted to remind everyone that next Monday is the deadline for the golf outing RSVP's. Even if you don't golf, please try to join us for the dinner portion of the day. It will be a fun night and we would love to see everyone there.

Be well
Rene & Alicia

Subject: Alicia Update June 10
Date: 6/10/03 3:11:20 PM Eastern Daylight Time

We finally got a beautiful day here in New York! It's warm, sunny and 81 degrees! Yeah! Everyone is doing well as we are winding down with all our school activities. Today was author's day for Alicia's class, a chance for the kids to read various works from the past year. It was very poignant when Alicia read her dedication to her second grade teacher. "I dedicate this book to my teacher for sending me home work so I wouldn't be left back!"; out of the mouths of babes. Unfortunately, with the excitement of the day and a bit too much snacking, I got a call to pick Alicia up by noon because she wasn't feeling well. That's ok, somebody to help me to plant flowers, except she is nowhere to be found. Seems my children mysteriously "disappear" when there is a project to be done! LOL

Due to incredible weather, we will be partying, hanging out with friends and hot tubbing tonight . . . Just in case it turns cold and rains tomorrow LOL.

Everyone stay well and enjoy!
Rene & Alicia

PS. Dear nurses; I have a feeling that we missed a clinic visit and port access . . . I didn't get a call . . . remember all those new rules to keep me in check? Well I hate to tell you this, but clinic visits are NOT on the top of our list . . . so let me know (we'll be in after school finishes)

Subject: Alicia Update June 19
Date: 6/19/03 11:44:54 PM Eastern Daylight Time

It's the end of the school year, hard to believe. Lauren finished up with her finals today and took the Earth Science Regent and now just has her school dance tomorrow night and graduation Monday night. J.J. and Alicia finish up their last full day tomorrow (a day of picnics and parties) and J.J. graduates Monday morning. In between the two graduations on Monday, we will fit in a clinic visit to have the former cancer patient get accessed and get checked.

I have to admit, I find it so enjoyable to watch Alicia be excited about school and all the excitement around the end of the year. I can't help but look at her and wonder why she has been through so much for such a young life. When I see how much joy she gets from everything though, I know deep in my heart that she really is enjoying each and everyday! She is a gem!

J.J. has a hockey tournament in New Jersey and we will let you know how clinic goes on Monday.

Have a great weekend and be well!
Rene & Alicia

RENE A. FESLER

Subject: Alicia Update June 23
Date: 6/23/03 2:27:38 PM Eastern Daylight Time

The rain has finally stopped here and there is a big yellow amd orange ball in the sky . . . I think they call it SUN! After a weekend of torrential rain it is a pleasure to feel some warmth. J.J. won his ice hockey tournament this weekend, which was a first for his team.

J.J. graduated this morning, Lauren is graduating this evening and we did a clinic visit in between. It is now very difficult to get Alicia up to the hospital because the prospect of being accessed is not so easy for her. She has been feeling fine, although they are carefully watching her spine now as her shoulders are growing uneven. This can be attributed directly to the radiation of her spine, but I guess in the scheme of things if she develops scoliosis, that's the least of our worries. Next month they will look again and possibly refer her to an orthopedist. Next week she has a CAT scan and an MRI.

Life is busy, but life is good!

> *Hope everyone is doing well . . .*
> *Rene & Alicia*

Subject: Alicia Update Happy 4ᵗʰ of July!
Date: 7/4/03 10:46:03 AM Eastern Daylight Time

Wishing everyone a Happy 4ᵗʰ! Time sure seems to be flying (guess this is a sign of growing older); Alicia has been feeling good and enjoying herself swimming, bicycle riding, kickball and movies. Her hair has grown back to a point that she will go out without a bandana and is feeling confident that she looks like every other kid.

Lauren started her round of sports camps at St. Anthony's and J.J. and Alicia have been enjoying just spending time together. I love watching the two of them playing golf on the front lawn or hear them just talking to each other about what they should play, instead of what it feels like to be on chemotherapy. Alicia and her friends have put together a memory book documenting their lives and what they mean to each other. It is very poignant and looking through the photos of the past year; it is sobering to me just how sick Alicia really looked. Looking back at these photos made me a bit reflective and brought up a lot of scary thoughts of what life has been like for us. I have to be totally honest; post treatment is more unsettling than being on treatment. I guess when we were following the doctors orders, I felt as though I was proactive, actively fighting the cancer and really didn't think about it. Now being off chemotherapy, I can't help but wonder, "Is she ok?" It is a very unsettling feeling, and I am hoping and praying that I will one day not feel so vulnerable and helpless against this dreaded disease.

Well enough with my psychoanalysis . . . I am a bit stressed over the golf outing which is two weeks away. I want to thank all of you who are volunteering and for offering your assistance.

Enjoy your day, and keep it safe with any fireworks you may have!

God Bless America and all of you!
Rene & Alicia

Subject: Alicia Update July 16
Date: 7/16/03 4:23:51 PM Eastern Daylight Time

Being forthright has been one of those qualities about me that you either "love" or "hate." Throughout the past year, I have taken a no holds barred approach to cancer, treatment and the psychological aspect of it all. Whether it was the right way or not to handle such an overwhelming situation, it worked for me and my kids and that's what mattered at the time. Well in all the hubbub of running this Foundation and trying to just put things back to normal, something along the line people forget that we are and always will be a cancer family. Cancer is not a broken bone that once mended is quickly forgotten. IT not only has a physical effect, there is a whole emotional effect that changes who you are and what your priorities are. I look at Alicia everyday and pray that her cancer will NEVER return. I also am reminded with every hospital visit and medical test we go to, just how fragile a little 7 year old can be and how unfair it is for a little child to have to endure such hardship. Today we went for an MRI and CAT scan, and while I am pleased to tell you that there is NO cancer evident, I can't help but share my disappointment that there are other issues that are a direct result of her treatment. These issues would most likely send a "regular" family to doctors in a panic, but we are a cancer family . . . wasn't that way until recently, but we will be for the rest of our lives, and we will take it in stride like everything else we do.

There is a reason the Foundation exists and people are working so hard to help us help others. Don't ever underestimate the trauma of cancer by thinking there is an end to it all, there is not. Never minimize the impact of cancer upon a family unless you have had the horrible

RENE A. FESLER

misfortune of experiencing it yourself. Children should NOT get cancer, yet they do. Because my little 7 year old named Alicia has suffered, we wish to help those who might not be so strong or so lucky. Count your blessings and make a difference in the lives of those around you. It shouldn't take a life threatening disease to appreciate what's truly important!

Be well
Rene & Alicia

Subject: Alicia Update July 23
Date: 7/23/03 11:53:12 AM Eastern Daylight Time

We went to clinic today and Alicia did great. She brought a friend with us and we needed to hurry back since I am babysitting her little sister for the day. She is a pleasure to watch and is so cute . . . she likes me, and when I find someone who does, I hold onto them like glue! LOL

For those who have not heard, the golf outing was a huge success! If you visit the website and click on events you can see pictures from the day; again a huge thank you to all our participants' sponsors and volunteers. We will have some down time for the next few weeks before we start gearing up for our next fundraising event, black tie cocktail party Monte Carlo night.

Alicia and I leave for Chicago tomorrow evening for a fundraising luncheon/silent auction on Saturday. Our dear friends the Konopasek family is hosting for us and we are very excited and honored to be attending. Keep an eye on the website for pictures of this event.

Hope everyone is doing well
Rene & Alicia

Subject: Alicia Update July 28
Date: 7/28/03 12:42:17 PM Eastern Daylight Time

Hope this Monday finds everyone well. Alicia and I just "blew" in from the windy city yesterday after attending a fundraiser that our friends the Konopasek family, were kind enough to host for the Foundation. It was a huge success and a lot of fun. Especially for Alicia and her friend Gennah who joined us with her dad Michael one of my board members, on this sojourn. We spent all Friday afternoon at the American Girls store in Chicago. There was a live show called "Circle of Friends" (I can't stop humming the tune) followed by "high tea." Finger sandwiches never tasted so good! We visited the John Hancock building observation deck (someone in our party thought it was the Sears tower LOL) and had an all around wonderful trip driving around Chicago. Anyone who has traveled with moi knows that one of the main requirements of any trip to "make a memory." This is when we stop for a moment and try to take a mental snapshot to look back upon. The past year we have had many memories . . . some better than others. It's nice to realize with the exciting week we have had, the memories are getting better!

Some serious money has been raised this past week that is being put to good use and I am truly astounded just how generous and helpful people are. It is such a testament to the goodness of people when there seems to be so much negative around. You all know how I thrive in a positive environment (no sourpusses allowed LOL) and feel so motivated by all that has been going on, that I am looking forward to our next event and the good we can do. Any of the fundraisers we do, while the main goal is to benefit the Foundation, they give any and every one who wants to an opportunity to participate. Not every event is for everyone, unless you are me LOL, but if you are going out for dinner anyway, why not do it with a bunch of friends for a worthy cause?

Hope everyone has had the opportunity to view the pictures from the golf outing, the Chicago ones will be online shortly.

Be well, stay positive and drop me a line to let me know how your summer is going!

Rene & Alicia

Subject: Alicia Update August 9
Date: 8/9/03 1:02:15 AM Eastern Daylight Time

Hope this email finds everyone well, hard to believe it is the middle of August already. Alicia is doing well, which is always a good thing to hear, God I hope and pray I never have to write an email otherwise, and it is Friday and the air conditioning upstairs has broken in the house. I have a family friend coming tomorrow morning to fix it, hopefully he can, but in the mean time you know what those children of mine needed to do? Figure out which neighbor has the coldest air conditioning and go stay at that house LOL. We had movie night on the driveway tonight, since some neighbors were upset that *the blonde has not been sitting out front lately. Do you think anyone else has a driveway that might be suitable? LOL and we needed to do a midnight Taco Bell run . . .*

Life is good and we are truly blessed, just taking things one day at a time. I hope everyone is focusing on what is important in life and not getting bogged down in nonsense and minutia. I have been spending time reading some of my past emails and trying NOT to cry . . . a scary journey the rawness of it all hit home. It is shocking to me after reading them just how sad and stressful the past year could have been. It seems that the blonde had more wisdom than I ever knew and a vision of our destiny. I am surprised by the strength that lurks within . . . Although I feel as though I am perched on the edge of some wonderful journey, I wonder if I might be ready to plummet into an abyss of sadness and self pity? It depends on ones perspective, my perspective. I choose the high road for cancer care, as a way to raise my kids and a way to live my life. It is a positive journey, it is a wonderful life!

LIFE AFTER CANCER

THERE WERE OTHER e-mails after this one, but this one seemed to sum it all up. It was like a closing chapter. What started out as a means of communicating to family and friends quickly turned into a memoir of our lives—a snapshot of a moment in time and a valuable lesson in adversity and our reaction to it. My e-mails taught a valuable lesson to many, and while today they provide a link to our past, they are a testament of who we are and how we got to where we are today.

My children are doing well. Alicia is doing well. Thank God, she has maintained her health and is a typical kid. She does have scoliosis due to her spinal surgery and radiation, but we are following it carefully under an orthopedist's watchful eye. This is a minor condition that we are dealing with and miniscule compared to what could have been. Her life, as with all of our lives, will never be the same, but I know for us life is better. Early on, I said that cancer can make you either bitter or better, the difference between the two lies with the letter *I* and what you do with it. How I handle myself, how I interact with others, and how I choose to live my life.

Life after cancer has not been easy, though, as relationships between all of us have changed. New friendships were forged, while older, more familiar ones seemed to fade away. There were those people I believed could not handle cancer's reality who showed strength and support beyond my wildest imagination. There were those who I believed to be strong who just seem to distance themselves from us, unable or unwilling to face our reality. That is okay, because we all have our own path and destiny. While I feel a twinge of sadness for those people who missed the deeper meaning in what was happening to us, that is what life is all about. Friendships that ebb and flow like the tide. We are blessed. Life is wonderful, and not a day goes by that I do not reflect on just how good it has been for us. The new friendships we have forged, the incredible memories we have made, and the opportunity to take something that could have been horrific and turned it into something positive not only for us, but for countless other kids with cancer. While I sometimes miss the innocence we had prior to Alicia's cancer, life has new meaning and direction. Her illness and her wishes have translated into helping others dealt a similar fate. God only gives you what you can handle, and I guess he gave us a bit more than most. I have no regrets for our past, just aspirations and dreams for our future—our wonderful future!

INDEX

A

Acyclovir 99 *see also* medications
admittance (*see also* hospital) 21,
    63-4, 66-7, 74, 82, 93, 111, 116,
    137-8
Alicia (cancer survivor)
  appetite 52
  back surgery 20, 24, 33, 83
  bone marrow transplant 97-8
  diagnosis 46, 96-7, 151-2
  treatment 16-42, 45-64, 66-7,
      70-1, 74-7, 81-6, 88-95, 97-8,
      100-1, 105-11, 113-14, 116-32,
      135-45, 148-50, 152-5, 158-68
anesthesia 61-2 *see also* medications
antibiotic 91 *see also* medications
Aranesp 49, 58, 77, 89, 103, 105,
    140
Aygun (oncologist) 60

B

backache 17, 122
blood counts 49, 61, 122
blood pressure 108-9, 117, 125
blood samples 39, 92
blue cell tumor 31
Bombeck, Erma
  "If I Had My Life to Live Over"
      146
bone pain 47
bone scan 19, 99-101, 109, 138, 162

C

cancer 14, 20, 30-1, 37, 41, 56, 79,
    96, 151, 166, 170
  kids 152 *see also* cancer patients
  survivor 154
  treatment 37, 56, 79 *see also*
      medications
  bone 96, 101, 125
cancer care 33, 37, 59, 139, 149, 169
cancer cells 56
cancer patients 14, 39, 41, 56, 70,
    128, 132, 164
cancer world 37, 107, 111, 118
CAT scan 62, 76, 99-101, 109, 138,
    140-1, 162, 165-6
Caulfield (Alicia's first-grade teacher)
    48, 60, 110-11, 124
Charlie (New York City firefighter/
    Maureen's husband) 51-2
chemo cycle 79, 95, 99, 103, 107,
    123, 127
chemotherapy (*see also* treatment
    under cancer) 39, 41, 56-7, 86,
    112-13, 116, 121, 124, 126,
    128, 136, 138, 152, 165-6
child-life specialist 59
Children's Cancer Center 110, 112,
    141
clinic
  visits 79, 164
crowning glory 39 *see also* hair loss

D

death (*see also* life)   14, 16, 39, 44, 68,
   98, 116, 119, 130, 149, 151-2
Denise (one of the operators)   66
disease   14, 32, 37, 40, 51, 70, 81,
   96, 166-7
Disney World   16
doctors *see individual names of doctors*
drugs   26, 86, 117 *see also*
   medications

E

e-mails   37, 43, 102, 114, 118, 139, 170
early intervention program   22
Earth Science Regent   164
echocardiogram   75, 91, 109, 140
emergency room   24 *see also* hospital
EMLA   39
etoposide   117

F

fever   47, 77, 98-9, 142
First Annual Honeysuckle Foundation
   for Children with Cancer Golf
   Classic   153
foundation   9, 121, 124, 133, 141,
   143-4, 149, 151, 153, 155,
   158-9, 161, 166-8
fundraising   71, 101, 124, 155, 167

G

Giacalone (*see also* Alicia, Lauren, *and*
   J. J.)   49, 92, 112, 123, 127,
   129, 135, 137, 140-2
growing pains   17

H

hair loss   39
Hersheypark   97
homeschooling   48-50, 52, 110
Honeysuckle Court   98, 117, 122,
   128, 154, 162
Honeysuckle Foundation for Children
   with Cancer   4, 9, 143, 153,
   159
hospital   20-1, 23-4, 28, 30-1, 33-5,
   41, 46, 48, 56, 59-60, 79, 82,
   92, 99-101, 107, 127
   bed   29
   protocol   30
   smell   33

I

If I Had My Life to Live Over
   (Bombeck)   146
injections   56-7, 61, 135

J

J. J. (Alicia's brother)   11, 16, 24,
   27-8, 35, 46, 81
Jingle Belle (puppy)   129, 132, 135-7,
   140, 145, 150
John (Alicia's doctor)   19-20

K

Kelly (nurse)   88
Konopasek family   167

L

Lauren (Alicia's sister)   7, 16, 27, 38,
     117, 119, 122, 125, 129, 162-5
leukemia   14, 97-8
Long Island Jewish Hospital   60-1
Louise (Alicia's handmade bunny)
     53

M

Maureen (Lauren's religious teacher)
     51-2, 101
medications   24, 39, 47-8, 56-7, 70,
     88-9, 109, 135, 137
Mediport (*see also* medications)   32,
     39, 41, 49, 61-2, 64, 75, 83,
     143, 152
Mittler (doctor)   20-1, 23, 31
MRI   19-20, 48, 100-1, 140-1, 162,
     165-6
Murphy's Law   65, 75
myringotomy   33 *see also* surgery

N

nausea   39, 47, 91, 136
Neupogen   48-9, 58, 95, 140 *see also*
     medications
Noreen (Rene and Alicia's friend, a
     cancer survivor)   70
North Shore Pediatric Cancer Center
     143
North Shore University Hospital   24
Novocain   39 *see also* medications

O

occupational therapy   22

P

parenting technique   28
pathology   31-2, 34
pediatric neurosurgeon   16, 20, 84
pediatric oncology   60, 97, 103, 153
pediatric ward   83-4
physical therapist   33, 36
platelet transfusion   92
Polly Pockets   23, 107, 117
prognosis   22, 98, 154 *see also*
     diagnosis *under* Alicia

R

radiation
     port verification   39, 56, 60-2,
          74-6, 79, 81-6, 88-91, 165, 170
     simulation   61
     therapy   60, 86
radiology   19, 60
recovery   33, 37
red cell production   89
red count (*see also* white count, blood
     count)   49, 58, 67, 77-8, 84-5,
     92, 103, 105, 140
rheumatoid arthritis   17

S

sensory integration difficulties   22
spinal surgery   22, 30, 170
spine   17, 19, 21, 60, 74, 76, 165
     alignment   76
steroids   21, 26, 29 *see also* medications
Stony Brook University Hospital   100
surgery 20-4, 28, 30-4, 83, 136, 154, 157-8, 170
symptoms   30, 88, 91 *see also* nausea,
     backache, hair loss, *and* growing pains

T

tonsillectomy   33 *see also* surgery

transfusion   39, 49-50, 61, 67, 70,
     77-9, 84-6, 92-3, 103, 105

tumor   20-1, 23, 30-1, 136

Tylenol   77, 89 *see also* medications

W

West Nile Virus   105

white count   58, 95, 140, 143

X

x-rays   76, 83, 91

LaVergne, TN USA
22 May 2010
183437LV00004BA/1/P